The Holistic Guide for Cancer Survivors

Mark Greener spent a decade in biomedical research before joining *MIMS Magazine* for GPs in 1989. Since then, he has written on health and biology for magazines worldwide for patients, healthcare professionals and scientists. He is a member of the Royal Society of Biology and is the author of 22 other books, including *The Heart Attack Survival Guide* (2012) and *The Holistic Health Handbook* (2013), both published by Sheldon Press.

Overcoming Common Problems Series

Selected titles

A full list of titles is available from Sheldon Press,
36 Causton Street, London SW1P 4ST and on our website at
www.sheldonpress.co.uk

Beating Insomnia: Without really trying
Dr Tim Cantopher

Cider Vinegar
Margaret Hills

Coeliac Disease: What you need to know
Alex Gazzola

Coping Successfully with Hiatus Hernia
Dr Tom Smith

**Coping with a Mental Health Crisis:
Seven steps to healing**
Catherine G. Lucas

Coping with Difficult Families
Dr Jane McGregor and Tim McGregor

Coping with Endometriosis
Jill Eckersley and Dr Zara Aziz

Coping with Headaches and Migraine
Alison Frith

Coping with Memory Problems
Dr Sallie Baxendale

Coping with Schizophrenia
Professor Kevin Gournay and Debbie Robson

Coping with the Psychological Effects of Illness
Dr Fran Smith, Dr Carina Eriksen
and Professor Robert Bor

Coping with Thyroid Disease
Mark Greener

Depression and Anxiety the Drug-Free Way
Mark Greener

Depressive Illness: The curse of the strong
Dr Tim Cantopher

Dr Dawn's Guide to Brain Health
Dr Dawn Harper

Dr Dawn's Guide to Digestive Health
Dr Dawn Harper

**Dr Dawn's Guide to Healthy Eating for
Diabetes**
Dr Dawn Harper

Dr Dawn's Guide to Healthy Eating for IBS
Dr Dawn Harper

Dr Dawn's Guide to Heart Health
Dr Dawn Harper

Dr Dawn's Guide to Sexual Health
Dr Dawn Harper

Dr Dawn's Guide to Toddler Health
Dr Dawn Harper

Dr Dawn's Guide to Weight and Diabetes
Dr Dawn Harper

Dr Dawn's Guide to Women's Health
Dr Dawn Harper

Dr Dawn's Guide to Your Baby's First Year
Dr Dawn Harper

The Fibromyalgia Healing Diet
Christine Craggs-Hinton

How to Stop Worrying
Dr Frank Tallis

**Invisible Illness: Coping with misunderstood
conditions**
Dr Megan A. Arroll and Professor
Christine P. Dancey

Living with Fibromyalgia
Christine Craggs-Hinton

Living with Hearing Loss
Dr Don McFerran, Lucy Handscomb
and Dr Cherilee Rutherford

**Living with the Challenges of Dementia:
A guide for family and friends**
Patrick McCurry

**Overcoming Emotional Abuse: Survive
and heal**
Susan Elliot-Wright

**Overcoming Low Self-esteem with
Mindfulness**
Deborah Ward

**Post-Traumatic Stress Disorder:
Recovery after accident and disaster**
Professor Kevin Gournay

The Stroke Survival Guide
Mark Greener

Ten Steps to Positive Living
Dr Windy Dryden

Treating Arthritis: The drug-free way
Margaret Hills and Christine Horner

Understanding High Blood Pressure
Dr Shahid Aziz and Dr Zara Aziz

**Understanding Yourself and Others:
Practical ideas from the world of coaching**
Bob Thomson

When Someone You Love Has Dementia
Susan Elliot-Wright

The Whole Person Recovery Handbook
Emma Drew

Overcoming Common Problems

The Holistic Guide for Cancer Survivors

MARK GREENER

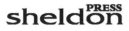

First published in Great Britain in 2016

Sheldon Press
36 Causton Street
London SW1P 4ST
www.sheldonpress.co.uk

British Library Cataloguing-in-Publication Data
A catalogue record for this book is available from the British Library

ISBN 978-1-84709-332-5
eBook ISBN 978-1-84709-333-2

Typeset by Fakenham Prepress Solutions, Fakenham, Norfolk NR21 8NN
First printed in Great Britain by Ashford Colour Press
Subsequently digitally reprinted in Great Britain

eBook by Fakenham Prepress Solutions, Fakenham, Norfolk NR21 8NN
Produced on paper from sustainable forests

To Ophelia, Yasmin, Rory and Rose, with love

Contents

A note to the reader

This is not a medical book and is not intended to replace advice from your doctor. Consult your pharmacist or doctor if you believe you have any of the symptoms described, and if you think you might need medical help.

Introduction

Every 100 seconds, someone, somewhere in the UK receives the devastating news that they have cancer. According to Cancer Research UK, doctors diagnosed 338,623 new cancers during 2011. Partly because we're living longer, half the population of the UK will probably develop cancer at least once.[1] Some people develop two or more *primary* cancers.

Despite remarkable advances in screening, diagnosis and treatment, some people still regard cancer as a death sentence. Certainly, some malignancies deserve this reputation: just one in five adults with pancreatic cancer in England survives for at least a year, for example. And someone dies from cancer every three minutes or so: cancer claimed 161,823 lives during 2012.

Even though cancer mortality rates have fallen by almost 10 per cent over 10 years in the UK, according to Cancer Research UK, the number of deaths continues to rise. In 2013, 1 person in every 352 in the UK died from cancer compared to 1 in 320 during 2003. Four-fifths of cancer deaths occur in people aged 65 and over. More than half of the deaths occur in those aged 75 years and older. So, as we're living longer, the number of people who die from cancer is increasing.

Nevertheless, more people than ever survive cancer or, if the disease proves incurable, live better for longer. In the 1970s, only one-quarter of people diagnosed with cancer survived for 10 years or more. Today, half survive for at least a decade.[1] For each woman diagnosed with breast cancer, 10 more have survived the malignancy.[2] In the UK, roughly two million people – about 1 in every 33 – are cancer survivors. Doctors expect this figure to reach four million by 2030.[1]

However, the advances in screening, diagnosis and treatment that underlie these improvements have left many cancer survivors facing long-term problems. Some problems don't arise until months or even years after cancer treatment ends, such as osteoporosis (brittle bone disease) following endocrine (hormonal) therapies, heart disease after certain types of chemotherapy or radiotherapy, and malignancies caused by the initial treatment.[1]

You and your family will also probably live with a considerable psychological and emotional burden. You may feel emotionally numb, uncertain, anxious and depressed. You might live in fear that the cancer will recur. You may feel conscious of your body image or have concerns about sexuality and fertility, discrimination, and relationships.[1] Some cancer survivors feel abandoned and isolated. After all, cancer teams inevitably focus on treating cancers rather than managing chronic problems or helping you adjust long term. Often families, friends and colleagues wonder what to say and do. This book aims to help you overcome these challenges and help you live a full and fulfilled life during and after your cancer treatment, even if your cancer can't be cured.

The cancer journey

Broadly, a person with cancer's journey takes place in three stages.

- Soon after diagnosis, the cancer team tries to cure or limit the damage to your body caused by the malignancy. This may involve surgery, radiotherapy, chemotherapy, hormonal treatments or, usually, a mixture of approaches. Although you may feel that your life is in your cancer team's hands, you can still deal with side effects, remain positive and keep your strength up. Don't underestimate the importance of these steps: they give the cancer treatment the best chance of working, help limit collateral damage and maximize your quality of life.
- During the recovery phase, you get over the worst effects of treatment and restore your physical and mental well-being. The cancer team will monitor you to detect and treat any relapses.
- During the maintenance phase, you take steps to prevent or delay a recurrence, prevent additional malignancies and reduce the risk of other preventable diseases, such as heart attacks, osteoporosis and strokes.[3]

In some ways, you're a survivor at any of these stages, not just if you receive the all clear. You can 'survive' treatment with, for example, the least impact on your life as possible. Indeed, some cancers are becoming chronic diseases. You might take hormone therapy for at least 5 years to lower the risk of breast cancer recurring, for example. You may take some other treatments for as long as the therapy holds the cancer in check. If the malignancy grows slowly and isn't causing symptoms – such as some prostate cancers – you may decide to delay treatment, but keep an eye on the tumour. Doctors call this *watchful waiting*.

During your cancer journey, you will see a range of healthcare professionals and receive high-tech treatments. Don't worry if you find the details difficult to understand at first. Some new treatments for cancer are very sophisticated and work on complex and complicated biological pathways inside cells. Some are at the very edge of our scientific understanding. Even non-specialist healthcare professionals can have difficulty understanding how they work. So, always ask your cancer team and patient groups, such as Cancer Research UK and Macmillan Cancer Support, if you don't understand something or have questions.

Complementary and alternative medicines

Despite using some of the most scientifically advanced drugs and devices, healthcare professionals caring for people with cancer are among the most open-minded about complementary and alternative medicines (CAMs). According to Cancer Research UK, up to a third of people with cancer use one or more CAMs at some time during their illness. Almost half of people with some malignancies, such as breast cancer, use CAMs. Many more may use CAMs, but never tell their cancer team.[4] (As we'll see, this isn't a good idea.) CAMs and lifestyle changes help many people. But, and I make no apologies for stressing this several times, CAMs and lifestyle changes support conventional therapies – they are not replacements.

CAMs and lifestyle changes help restore your sense of control over the cancer and your life more generally. It's easy to feel disempowered when you face cancer and that you can do little to improve your prospects. If this book has one message, it's that this simply isn't true. You can help alleviate or prevent side effects and take steps to live with cancer's symptoms.

Scientific studies suggest, for example, that aromatherapy may reduce the need for laxatives or painkillers.[4] Acupuncture can reduce nausea and vomiting, increase energy and physical activity in people receiving chemotherapy[5] and alleviate bladder discomfort following radiotherapy.[6] Adapting your diet can help deal with diarrhoea, constipation, nausea and vomiting. And, while it may be the last thing you feel like doing, exercise helps tackle cancer-related fatigue.

Partly because of this growing evidence, and partly because they could see the benefits, the attitude of many cancer teams towards CAMs changed. Initially, many conventional doctors and nurses viewed CAMs with scepticism if not outright hostility. This gradually softened into a grudging acceptance. Today, increasingly, CAMs form part of the cancer treatment plan. In some countries, such as China and Vietnam, the same doctor may offer complementary and conventional medicine.[7] In the UK, complementary and conventional medicine run in parallel. Nevertheless, cancer centres increasingly combine CAMs and conventional treatments, so-called integrative oncology. As this shows, you need to take a holistic approach that integrates conventional medicines, CAMs and lifestyle changes.

Tragically, however, some alternative practitioners suggest stopping conventional therapy and use their approach to 'cure' cancer, often based on a couple of spectacular *spontaneous remissions*. The overwhelming majority of alternative practitioners are well-meaning, kind, honest people who firmly believe that their therapy works. A few are frauds, charlatans and confidence tricksters. (Mind you, some healthcare professionals are far from perfect.) But never believe claims that they can cure cancer when conventional medicine cannot. Never stop conventional treatment. And be cautious if a practitioner only highlights one or two remarkable improvements. If it sounds too good to be true, it probably is.

A personal journey

The bravery that most people show when they face cancer never ceases to amaze and inspire me. Nevertheless, your cancer journey is deeply personal, often difficult and at times frightening. I hope that the suggestions in this book will make life a little easier for you and your family. I am afraid, however, that there are no guarantees.

Cancer is an enigmatic, capricious, unpredictable disease. Despite advances in imaging and genetics no-one can precisely define your prognosis. No-one can accurately predict the severity of your side effects or the long-term complications you'll experience. No-one can forecast with certainty the disruption to your life the cancer and its treatment will cause. Your cancer team offers educated guesses based on scientific data: but there are countless cases where patients defied their doctor's expectations.

Similarly, no-one can guarantee that the suggestions in the book will definitely work for you. This book offers general information and suggestions that do not replace the advice from your cancer team, which is tailored to you, your cancer and your circumstances. Always contact your GP or cancer team if you feel unwell or think that your disease is getting worse, even if it's between appointments. I wish you all the best.

A note about references

It's impossible to cite all the numerous medical and scientific studies used to write this book. (Apologies to anyone whose work I missed.) I've highlighted certain papers to illustrate important points and themes. You can find a summary by entering the details here: <www.ncbi.nlm.nih.gov/pubmed>. Some full papers are available online free or at a reduced rate for patients. Larger libraries might stock or allow you to access some medical journals. Some of the papers may seem rather erudite if you do not have a medical or biological background. But don't let that put you off. If you feel you don't understand something please ask your GP, pharmacist, cancer team or a helpline run by a charity.

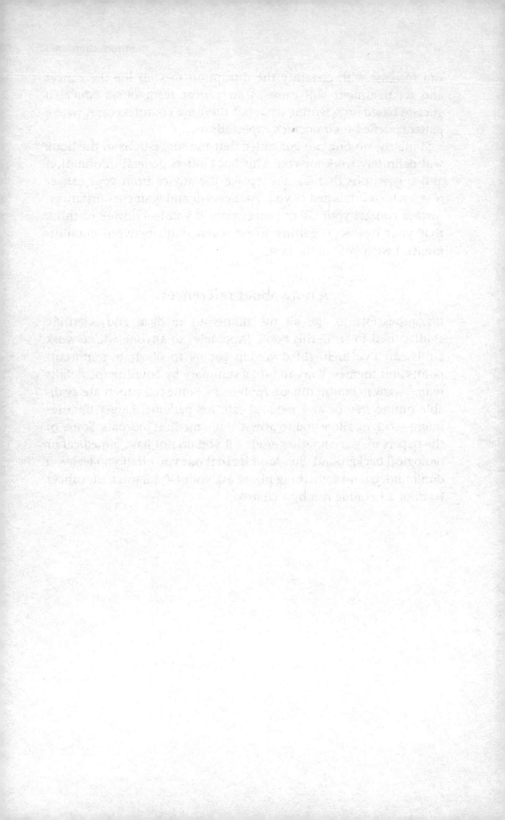

1

Understanding the 'Big C'

I'm not, as my wife reminds me regularly, the same man I was a few years ago. Literally. I shed about 30,000 skin cells and make about 300 million blood cells a minute. My cells live, on average, for 7 to 10 years, although this varies from about four months for my red blood cells to more than 50 years for some of my heart cells. I constantly repair, renew and replenish even my relatively long-lived cells: I replace the water in my body over a few weeks, for instance.[8]

We produce new cells to replace old and damaged tissues. Too few or too many cells can undermine an organ's or tissue's normal function. So, a finely balanced system of checks and balances controls cells' destruction and production. The immune system – which protects us from invading bacteria, viruses and parasites – destroys some damaged cells, for example. We also produce a cocktail of chemical messengers. Some promote cell division. Some reduce cell division. Some trigger cells to self-destruct. Such checks and balances mean that, when we're healthy, the number of cells we produce balances the numbers we lose.

Different cancers unbalance this system in different ways. Some cancers stop the immune system from destroying the malignancy. In some cancers, the messengers no longer stimulate worn out cells to self-destruct. In other malignancies, the person produces more cells than they destroy.

Cancer cells are profoundly abnormal and no longer perform their normal functions. As the cancer grows, abnormal malignant cells replace more and more of the healthy tissue. Eventually, the organ cannot compensate. So, symptoms emerge and the organ begins to fail. That's why, unfortunately, untreated cancers can eventually kill.

Cells, tissues and organs

Cells are your body's building blocks. A bacterium, spermatozoa, ovum (egg) and the amoeba you may remember from biology class are all single cells. You need a microscope to see most single cells.

An organ is a self-contained, organized collection of cells with one or more functions. The lungs are collection of cells that exchange toxic carbon dioxide for the oxygen that keeps us alive. The liver is a collection of cells that, among other actions, removes waste. The heart is a collection of cells that pumps blood. A tissue bridges the gap between a cell and an organ. Most organs consist of several tissues.

Hundreds of cancers

We replenish, repair and renew every part of our body. So, cells in any part of our body can turn cancerous. Indeed, oncologists – doctors who study cancer – recognize more than 200 malignancies. Some rare cancers emerge in only a handful of people each year. On the other hand, malignancies of the breast, lung, prostate and bowel account for about half of cancers (54 per cent) and cancer deaths (46 per cent).

To complicate matters, the same cancer's characteristics can differ dramatically from person to person. There are at least four main subtypes of breast cancer, for instance, each caused by different abnormalities[9] and each with a different prognosis (outlook) and sometimes treatment. Cancers also vary depending on their cell or tissue of origin. Basal cell carcinoma, squamous cell carcinoma, melanoma and Merkel cell carcinoma are all skin cancers, but arise from different cells. So, they have different characteristics, prognoses and treatments.

A tumour can evolve over time, which is one reason treatment may alter during your cancer journey. For these reasons, I doubt if there'll ever be a *single* cure for cancer. Based on our current knowledge of oncology (the study of cancer), you'll need different cures for different cancers, different cures for different people, and even different cures for the same cancer in the same person at different times. Indeed, some cancers can already be cured.

What's in a name?

Cancers tend to be named after their origin. Here are some examples.

- A thin layer of epithelial cells lines many parts of the body, including the skin, intestines and lungs. Carcinomas are cancers that arise from epithelial cells.
- Connective tissue, such as cartilage or bone supports, connects and separates other tissues and organs. Sarcomas refers to cancers in connective tissue.
- Lymphomas arise in lymph glands or other organs of the lymphatic system (page 6).
- Leukaemia refers to cancers of white blood cells, which normally protect us from infections. Blood cancers do not normally form solid tumours.
- Melanoma arises in cells that give our skin colour.

Primary and secondary cancers

Doctors call the original tumour the *primary cancer*. Tumours that spread from the original tumour to other parts of your body are *secondary cancers* or *metastases*. So, a doctor will refer to, for instance, metastatic prostate cancer. This begins in the prostate gland, the doughnut-shaped, walnut-sized bundle of tissue that lies just beneath a man's bladder. The urethra, the tube that carries urine and sperm to the penis tip, runs through the middle of the prostate gland. In metastatic prostate cancer, malignancies arise in other parts of the body, such as the bone, bladder, kidney, lungs or liver. Advanced cancer, in general, means a cure is, unfortunately, unlikely. Most people with advanced cancer have metastases.

Doctors distinguish *second primary cancers* from secondary cancers. A second primary cancer refers to a new primary cancer (in other words, not a metastasis) in a person who has already had a malignancy. So, a skin cancer caused by too much sun in a person who survived breast cancer is a second primary malignancy. At one meeting I attended, an oncologist mentioned that patients often find second primary cancers especially difficult to cope with. 'They feel that they've had their cancer,' he said.

Secondary primary cancers can emerge for various reasons, including some cancer treatments.[1] For example, patients younger than 40 years of age treated with radiotherapy or chemotherapy for Hodgkin's lymphoma, non-Hodgkin's lymphoma or testicular cancer are roughly four times more likely than the general public to develop a second primary cancer.[1]

In addition, many risk factors cause more than one malignancy. For example, smoking tobacco causes lung cancer and malignancies in the mouth, lips, nose and sinuses, voice box, throat, oesophagus, stomach, pancreas, kidney, bladder, uterus, cervix, colon and rectum, and ovary, as well as the blood cancer acute myeloid leukaemia.

Similarly, people with one skin cancer are at much higher risk of developing new malignancies on other parts of their skin. So, it's important to check yourself for, for example, moles, spots and other skin blemishes that are growing, bleeding, changing in appearance or never heal completely. Use mirrors, family members or take a selfie to see 'difficult to view' skin areas. Ask your GP or cancer team if you are not sure what to look for. The British Association of Dermatologists publishes information leaflets about watching for and preventing skin cancers (<www.bad.org.uk/for-the-public/patient-information-leaflets>).

As a final example, inherited genetic problems could result in more than one malignancy. For instance, people with Lynch syndrome have inherited mutations in at least five genes that repair damaged DNA. So, they are especially prone to develop colorectal cancer at an early age and are more likely than those without Lynch syndrome to develop cancers of the womb, ovary, small bowel, pancreas, gall bladder and bile duct, and urinary tract.[10]

Benign and cancerous tumours

An abnormal accumulation of cells – a tumour, also called a neoplasm – isn't always cancerous. Doctors call non-cancerous accumulations of cells *benign* tumours. Some benign tumours become massive. Indian surgeons removed a 57 kg (almost 9 stone) mucinous cystadenoma, a benign tumour of the ovaries, from a 55-year-old woman. The tumour had grown slowly: her abdomen began to look distended some 13 years before the operation. However, financial constraints and family issues meant she didn't see a doctor.[11]

Unlike cancers, benign tumours do not invade other tissues or spread to other parts of the body. When they're removed by surgeons, most benign tumours do not regrow and they rarely cause serious health problems. Sometimes, however, a benign tumour can press on a nearby area, which may cause symptoms. An acoustic neuroma, for example, arises in the nerve from the ear to the brain and can cause problems with hearing and balance.[4]

Cancers, in contrast, are malignant – sometimes called invasive. In other words, the cancer can spread into (invade) nearby tissues. The term cancer comes from a Greek word meaning crab, which ancient healers felt described the appearance of the tumour and its blood vessels as it spread into the surrounding tissue.[12]

Spreading cancer around the body

Cells can break off from the cancer and travel in the blood or lymph system. These circulating cancer cells are malignant seeds. They can lodge in another tissue and, if the conditions are right, grow into a metastasis. Breast cancer, for example, typically metastases into the bone, liver and lung. Sometimes, the cancer has spread to other parts of the body by the time doctors diagnose the malignancy. Your prospects are worse if you're diagnosed with advanced cancer than with a small localized tumour that surgeons can remove easily. That's why screening, or seeing your GP as soon as you notice a lump or experience an 'alarm' symptom (page 13), is so important.

Your symptoms and prognosis depend on where metastases form. Symptoms of a lung metastasis differ from secondary cancer in the liver, for example. In one study, about three-quarters (73 per cent) of women with breast cancer and a single metastasis in their skeleton survived for 5 years. This compared with just over a fifth (22 per cent) of those with a metastasis in an internal organ, such as the liver or lung.[13]

The metastasis changes as it adapts to the new organ. But the metastasis retains many characteristics of the primary cancer. So, a liver metastasis is different to a primary liver cancer. However, liver metastasis from a breast cancer may also differ from its primary cancer. All this makes treatment of advanced cancer very complicated.

> ### What is lymph?
>
> Lymph is a clear, milky or yellowish fluid that bathes our tissues and contains white blood cells. That's why your lymph nodes (such as the glands under your chin and in your armpits) may swell when you have an infection or you're fighting cancer. Your lymph glands may also swell as invading cancer cells grow inside the node. So, the cancer team may remove or irradiate (treat with radiotherapy) lymph nodes near the cancer.

A cancer's development

Most primary cancers have been growing for years, even decades, before symptoms emerge. For example, liver disease can progress from hepatitis (liver inflammation) to cirrhosis (scarring) to cancer. But this takes typically takes 20–40 years. Cells divide into two 'daughter' cells. On average, a breast cancer cell divides every 100 days. A 1 cm breast cancer, the size that you might be able to feel or see on a mammogram, contains about a million cells.[2] It's probably been growing for between 5 and 6 years.

Screening can catch curable cancers

Screening aims to detect and treat cervical, breast, prostate and some intestinal cancers before they are large enough to undermine your health and well-being or to spread to other parts of the body. Early detection and rapid treatment offers the best prospect of a cure: surgeons can remove small localized cancers.

Screening can catch abnormal cells before they turn cancerous. Cancers don't emerge fully formed. Usually, the transformation of a healthy cell into a cancer begins when the number of cells in an organ or tissue increases. These cells appear normal under a microscope. Doctors call this hyperplasia. Over time, the cells begin to look abnormal, but not cancerous – which doctors call dysplasia. Hyperplasia and dysplasia do not always develop into cancer. Sometimes hyperplasia and dysplasia don't progress further. Sometimes the body's innate healing abilities restore normal healthy tissue. However, dysplastic cells can develop into a malignancy (Figure 1).

Cervical cancer screening, for example, aims to detect abnormal cells on the surface of the cervix (the neck of the womb at the

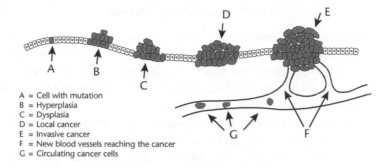

A = Cell with mutation
B = Hyperplasia
C = Dysplasia
D = Local cancer
E = Invasive cancer
F = New blood vessels reaching the cancer
G = Circulating cancer cells

Figure 1 The development of cancer

top of the vagina) before these become malignant. Doctors grade these abnormal cells – called *cervical intra-epithelial neoplasia* (CIN) – on a scale of 1 to 3, based on how abnormal the cells look under the microscope and how much of the cervix is affected. CIN isn't cancer. Over time, however, between two and three in every five CIN-2 (moderately abnormal) changes return to normal without treatment.[14] Unfortunately, doctors cannot yet predict which CINs will develop into cervical cancers. That's why every woman should attend for screening. Unfortunately, there are no screening tests for many deadly cancers – such as lung, ovary, brain or pancreas – although researchers are working on them.

How effective is screening?

Screening detects about 3 in 10 breast cancers and 1 in 20 colorectal (bowel) cancers.[1] Cancer Research UK found that of those colorectal cancers picked up by screening in England during 2012 and 2013, 37 per cent were caught at the earliest stage (stage 1) while 8 per cent were advanced malignancies (stage 4). This compares to 6 per cent and 40 per cent at stage 1 and 4 respectively for colorectal cancers diagnosed as emergencies and 18 per cent and 22 per cent of those diagnosed after the GP referred the patient to a specialist. To look at the figures another way, breast cancer mortality in the USA declined by almost a quarter (24 per cent) between 1990 and 2005. A statistical analysis found that improvements in chemotherapy accounted for half the improvement and screening for the remainder.[12]

Cancer's countless causes

With all the scare stories that regularly reach the headlines, you could be forgiven for thinking that almost anything can cause cancer. After all, over the years, studies have linked cancer to chemicals in food, toys and make up; air travel; bacon and sausages; sex . . . the list goes on, and on, and on.

There's usually something to these scare stories. Hundreds of chemicals are proven or likely to cause cancer in cells grown in the laboratory or experimental animals, at least. How this applies to our lives is, however, debatable. The higher you travel in the atmosphere the greater your exposure to cancer-causing cosmic rays. Processed and, probably, red meat seem to increase the risk of developing certain malignancies (page 48). And sex can spread cancer-causing infections. Indeed, infections cause about 1 in 27 cancers in the UK.[15] Human papilloma virus (HPV), for example, is responsible for most cervical cancers. You can catch HPV, which can also cause cervical and some head and neck cancers, through intercourse, oral sex or sharing sex toys, even after cleaning.[16, 17] Some hepatitis viruses can lead to liver cancer and can also spread through sex. You cannot, however, directly catch cancer.

On the other hand, a healthy lifestyle could prevent about two in every five cancers in the UK. In 2010, for example:

- tobacco smoking caused about 1 in 5 new cancers;
- in men, low intake of fruits and vegetables accounted for about 1 in 16 cancers;
- occupational exposures and alcohol consumption each accounted for about 1 in 20 cancers in men;
- in women, overweight and obesity accounted for about 1 in 14 cancers.[15]

Some risk factors are additive. The combination of excessive alcohol and smoking is more carcinogenic than either alone.[15] So, how do such diverse risk factors cause cancer? Usually, the answer is in your genes.

Radiation and cancer

In 1895, the German scientist Wilhelm Conrad Röntgen accidentally discovered X-rays while experimenting with vacuum tubes. A week later, Röntgen took the first radiograph, of his wife's hand, showing her bones and wedding ring. However, the radiographic pioneers soon realized that X-rays can cause burns and skin reactions. Then, in 1902, an X-ray technician developed a skin sore. This evolved into the cancer on his hand that killed him four years later.[18, 19] The first reports of leukaemia among people working with radioactive materials emerged in 1911.[19] Radiation destroyed the bone marrow of Marie Curie, who won two Nobel Prizes for her pioneering work on radioactive material, leaving her permanently anaemic. She died from leukaemia in 1934.[12]

Today, exposure to radioactive material (which scientists call ionizing radiation) probably causes about 1 in 50 cancers in the UK. The figures are higher for leukaemias: radiation causes about 1 in 13 leukaemias in women and 1 in 15 in men.[19]

Radon gas, produced from uranium in the earth, accounts for about half our total exposure to radiation. (You can learn more, including your local levels, at <www.ukradon.org>.) Other natural sources (including cosmic rays) account for about a third (35 per cent). Radiation received during diagnosis and medical procedures (excluding radiotherapy) account for most of the remainder (15 per cent).[19]

Genes and cancer

Almost every one of the trillions of cells in your body contains an 'instruction manual' to make your entire body, contained in DNA's famous double helix. The amount of DNA in your body never ceases to amaze me. Pulled into a single, microscopically thin strand, your DNA would go from Earth to the Sun and back more than 300 times, or wrap around the Earth's equator 2.5 million times.[20] DNA is tightly packed into 23 chromosomes that contain the 25,000 or so genes that determine your natural hair and skin colour, influence your height and weight, and build biological pathways that keep cells alive and working normally.

Genes tell cells what to do and when, such as when to divide and when to stop. In most cancers, these genetic instructions become corrupted (mutated). On average, we have between 40 and 60 genetic abnormalities. But not all mutations cause disease. Most mutations don't change the gene's meaning or the body can compensate – so the genetic abnormality doesn't matter. But some mutations alter the instruction and, in turn, how the cell works.[4]

Currently, biologists have identified around 100 genes that when mutated predispose to at least one cancer.[10] Some of these genes lead to cancer when they become inappropriately activated – it's almost as if the mutation presses the cell's accelerator to the floor. Some lead to cancer when they're blocked. These tumour suppressor genes slow cell division: the mutation takes the brake off the cell's division.[12] So, the cell divides over and over again.

Lifestyle factors, inherited genes and quality control errors

Many lifestyle factors linked to cancer – such as smoking, cancer-causing (carcinogenic) chemicals and excessive exposure to sunlight or tanning beds – can mutate genes. Everyone has 'healthy versions' of the genes linked to lung cancer: they ensure our cells divide normally. But carcinogens in smoke can mutate these genes. That's one reason why the risk of lung cancer is higher in smokers.[12] Cigarette smoke, for example, contains a chemical called benzopyrene, which binds to and damages DNA. Because of the ongoing DNA damage, continuing to smoke after a diagnosis of cancer can promote the malignancy's growth and metastases.[4]

You can also inherit mutated genes from your parents. That's why some malignancies – so-called *hereditary cancers* – run in families. Researchers have identified more than 50 mutated genes involved in hereditary cancers.[10] For example, about 1 in 100 women carry a gene – such as *BRCA1* or *BRCA2* – that dramatically increases their risk of developing breast, ovarian and perhaps some other cancers.[2, 21] Between 50 per cent and 80 per cent of women with an inherited mutation in *BRCA1* develop breast cancer, which is 3–5 times higher than the risk in women without these mutations.[12] *BRCA* genes seem to be involved in pathways that recognize and repair DNA damage.[21]

People with a skin disease called xeroderma pigmentosum also have defects in genes that control DNA repair, which they inherited from their parents. These people are very sensitive to the sun and are especially likely to develop skin cancers.[22]

Mutations can also arise from errors in the cell's quality control. Considering our cells divide trillions of times, they make remarkably few errors. The cell has numerous processes to check and repair mistakes. But sometimes these quality control mechanisms miss one – a bit like an editor missing a *speling* mistake in a book. That's one reason why most cancers become more common as we get older.[2] Errors made copying DNA accumulate over time. Older people have been also exposed to carcinogens and unhealthy lifestyles for longer. Meanwhile, we're less able to repair damaged cells as we get older. So, we accumulate DNA damage as we age.

Cancers are genetically unstable

Cancers are genetically unstable. So, the longer the cancer survives the greater the number of mutations that are likely to develop. A cancer probably accumulates six or seven critical mutations between the initial change and metastasis. Each mutation marks another step in the cancer's development (Figure 2).

One critical mutation may result in hyperplasia. Another may lead to the formation of the early, localized cancer. Another to metastasis. Another may mean that the cancer becomes resistant to a particular treatment – a bit like a bacterium becomes a super-bug after evolving resistance to an antibiotic. The cancer continues to divide – and increase in size – between the development of each of these critical mutations.[22]

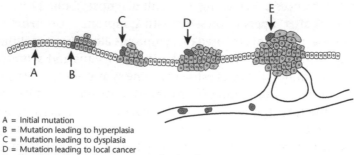

A = Initial mutation
B = Mutation leading to hyperplasia
C = Mutation leading to dysplasia
D = Mutation leading to local cancer
E = Mutation leading to invasive cancer and metastasis

Figure 2 Critical mutations in the development of cancer

This genetic instability means that the cancer accumulates numerous *passenger mutations*, which don't seem to influence the tumour's progression or the response to treatment. Sorting out which mutations drive the malignancy's growth, which influence the effectiveness of treatment, and which could lead to new screening techniques and therapeutic targets is one of the most promising and active areas in cancer research.

Communication breakdown

Genetic changes are not the only explanation for some cancer's development. For example, certain cancers could arise following interruptions to the flow of chemical signals that carry messages between nearby cells. This communication breakdown could disrupt the tissue's organization and development. Genetic changes might be a by-product of the disrupted organization caused by abnormal signalling.[22]

Mechanical forces also influence tissue development. For instance, mechanical forces during development form the finger-like villi that increases the surface area of your gut between 60 and 120 fold.[22] Estimates vary, but the folds could pack the equivalent of half a badminton court to a tennis court into your gut.[23] The viscosity (thickness) of your blood influences blood vessels' development.[22] Abnormal mechanical forces could drive the development of certain malignancies. Of course, more than one mechanism could contribute, perhaps at different stages in the cancer's development.

Diagnosing cancer

Despite advances in screening, GPs still diagnose about 17 in every 20 cancers after a person presents with symptoms.[1] Unfortunately, diagnosing most cancers based on symptoms alone is often difficult.

Each cancer produces a different pattern of signs and symptoms. And many 'minor' illnesses cause the same symptoms as potentially deadly cancers.[1] Indigestion (heart burn), headaches and backache may be the first sign of gastric (oesophageal or stomach), brain or pancreatic cancer respectively. But they are much more likely to be the symptoms of a poor diet, dehydration or a pulled muscle. Nevertheless, you should see your GP if the symptom persists. Public Health England, for instance, suggests that people who have

Table 1 Alarm symptoms for cancer

- Blood in your stools or urine
- Cough that lasts longer than 3 weeks
- Coughing up blood or blood-stained mucous
- Diarrhoea that lasts longer than 3 weeks
- Indigestion that lasts longer than 3 weeks or that is not relieved by medicines, such as antacids, bought without a prescription
- Lump, such as in the breast or testicle, or changes in the way they feel
- Rectal bleeding
- Swallowing problems (dysphagia)
- Unintentional weight loss

Based on Badenhorst J, Husband A, Ling J, et al.[24]

indigestion most days for three weeks or more should see their GP. Always see your GP if you have an alarm symptom (Table 1).

Because of the difficulty in diagnosing cancer based on symptoms alone, there is often a delay before the GP refers a person with suspected cancer to a specialist. The length of the delay depends on the cancer. More than nine in every ten patients with malignancies that produce characteristic symptoms or signs (e.g., breast cancer and melanoma) see a specialist after one or two GP consultations. For malignancies with less distinctive symptoms (e.g., lung cancer, myeloma and pancreatic cancer) at least a third of patients have three or more GP consultations before being referred.[1] So, if you are worried, don't be afraid to press your point and insist on a referral.

Viewing cancers

Doctors can take a peek inside your body in various ways to see if a tumour might account for your symptoms. They may use ultrasound and X-rays, for example. They may use a flexible camera called an endoscope. And they may use CT (computed tomography; sometimes called CAT – computerized axial tomography) and MRI (magnetic resonance imaging) scans, which can visualize the inside of your body in often awe-inspiring detail.

CT uses X-rays to produce numerous (often more than a hundred) 'slices' through your body. The beam varies in width, depending on the detail needed, from 1 mm to 10 mm. A computer rebuilds the slices into a single three-dimensional image in remarkably high resolution. In some cases, radiologists use a *contrast medium* to enhance fine detail. MRI uses powerful magnetic fields to provide an even more detailed view than CT.

Doctors will also probably run blood tests and look at a small sample of the tumour or tissue (a biopsy) under a microscope. They may test the sample to, for example, identify the genetic fingerprint. As we'll see in the next chapter, this can have a big impact on the choice of treatment for some cancers. They may also take biopsy of surrounding tissue (the margin) to see if the cancer has spread or to ensure it's all been removed during surgery.

2
Conventional cancer treatments

It's easy to forget just how much the prospects for people with many cancers have changed. In 1878, doctors in Vienna reported that only 1 in 20 women lived for three years after undergoing surgery for breast cancer.[18] Modern drugs, radiotherapy and surgery mean that about three-quarters of women with breast cancer now survive for at least 10 years.[4]

Tragically, however, even with sophisticated modern care, most advanced and metastatic cancers remain incurable.[4] Nevertheless, there are grounds for cautious optimism. In the early 1970s, 19 of every 20 men with metastatic testicular cancers died, usually within 1 year of diagnosis, according to the National Institutes of Health (NIH). Modern treatments cure four in five metastatic testicular cancers. Even if you have an advanced malignancy, the cancer team can help you live life to the fullest extent possible, for as long as possible.

Individualizing treatment

Each cancer in each patient is unique. So, the cancer team individualizes treatment depending on, for instance, the following factors.

- Your general health and well-being, which doctors call *performance status*. If you are fitter and stronger, you may be able to tolerate more 'aggressive' treatment with more side effects and a better chance of a good outcome than someone who is more frail.
- Your goals, plans and attitudes. Some people with metastatic cancer trade a few weeks or months of expected survival for what they see as a better quality of life if they don't experience side effects. Some men with metastatic prostate cancer are very concerned about losing sexual function, a common side effect of some treatments for this malignancy. So, they may refuse surgery

or certain drugs that could prolong their survival, but that may compromise sexual function.

- The site of the secondary tumours and your symptoms. Surgeons may be able to remove a tumour that causes pain because it presses on a nerve, bone or the spinal cord, for example. It's much harder to remove a brain tumour.
- The treatments (especially drugs) you've received before. Cancers can become resistant to a particular treatment. So, a drug used to treat the primary cancer might not work as well if it or a similar medicine is used to treat metastases.

Ensuring that management is right for you is one reason why it's so important to have a full and frank discussion with your cancer team before you embark on a course of treatment. It's worth exploring the uncertainties. So, if a doctor says you'll gain an expected year of life, you may benefit more or less than this. You may not develop the expected side effects, or they may be unexpectedly severe. A surgeon can't guarantee to cure a cancer – so they'll speak about 'curative intent'.

This book isn't intended to offer a comprehensive overview of conventional cancer treatments: there are far too many to discuss and oncology advances extremely quickly. This chapter briefly outlines the broad approaches. For more details about your specific treatment, speak to your cancer team or a charity such as Macmillan Cancer Support or Cancer Research UK. Their websites are invaluable sources of up-to-date information.

Lines of treatment

Most people with cancer need more than one treatment. Your initial management plan – the so-called first-line treatment – may include surgery, chemotherapy and radiotherapy. If the cancer recurs or doesn't respond adequately, you'll move to second-line treatment. If second-line treatment fails, you'll move to the third-line treatment and so on. The large number of drugs for some cancers means that you could have multiple lines: some women with breast cancer receive ten or more lines of treatment, for example.

Neoadjuvant and adjuvant therapy

Your cancer team may suggest neoadjuvant therapy, adjuvant treatment or chemoradiotherapy to increase the chances of a good outcome.

- Neoadjuvant therapy uses drugs to reduce the size of the tumour before radiotherapy or surgery.
- During adjuvant therapy, you take cancer drugs after radiotherapy or surgery to try to mop up any remaining small tumours and circulating cancer cells.
- During chemoradiotherapy, you receive a combination of radiotherapy and chemotherapy. The combination seems to kill malignant cells more effectively than either alone, possibly because the chemotherapy makes cancer cells more sensitive to radiation.

Surgery

Sometimes surgery is the only treatment you'll need. A surgeon can remove a localized malignancy that has not spread and, in so doing, cure the cancer. Obviously, small cancers are easier to remove than larger tumours. So, removing a small cancer is less likely to damage the surrounding area and often produces a better cosmetic outcome than an operation for a larger tumour. On the other hand, certain cancers, such as certain primary tumours and metastases in the brain, may be unsuitable for surgery.

The surgeon will send a sample of the cancer for tests, which helps decide if you need further surgery and any next steps in treatment. Usually, the surgeon removes some of the surrounding healthy tissue (the 'margin') or nearby lymph nodes. The lab will test the margin or the lymph nodes to ensure that the surgeon removed all the cancer.

Some people undergo surgery to remove *precancerous* lesions, such as small masses of cells called polyps in the stomach or intestine. (Lesions are areas of cells damaged by disease or injury.) Some polyps can develop into gastrointestinal cancer. Similarly, surgeons remove abnormal, precancerous areas of the cervix to prevent cervical cancer.

Other possible roles for surgery include the following.

- Preventing cancer. Some people at very high risk decide to remove their breasts, ovaries or parts of their bowel before pre-cancerous changes emerge.
- Reconstructive surgery to repair damage from an operation to remove the cancer or because the malignancy affected a visible part of the body. Advances in cosmetic surgery now mean that most people can achieve a good appearance, often despite extensive operations.
- Treating recurrences and metastases. A surgeon might be able to remove some or all secondary cancers, such as one or two liver metastases.
- Alleviating problems in advanced cancer. For example, a cancer may block the intestine. Surgery can bypass the blockage or allow the bowel to drain into a colostomy bag outside your body. Surgeons may insert feeding tubes if you are having difficulty eating.

The operation and the associated risks depend on, for example, the cancer, your particular symptoms and your performance status. So, discuss the risks and benefits with your cancer team and check out the information provided by patient support groups.

Chemotherapy

Chemotherapy – drugs that kill cells – can cure a few cancers. A combination of several drugs cures about 19 in every 20 testicular cancers, according to the NIH. The chemotherapy drug vincristine improved the chances of surviving childhood leukaemia from less than one in ten (10 per cent) in 1960 to more than nine in ten (90 per cent) today. More commonly, however, chemotherapy is one element in a planned programme of treatment. So, you might receive neoadjuvant or adjuvant chemotherapy.

Chemotherapy can also shrink metastases, which alleviates symptoms. That's one reason why, despite a reputation for side effects, chemotherapy often improves quality of life. The TAX 327 study, for instance, compared two chemotherapy drugs – docetaxel and mitoxantrone, both given with prednisone (which reduces the risk of allergic side effects) – for advanced prostate cancer when hormone treatments (see below) no longer worked. About one in five men (22–23 per cent) reported improved quality of life with docetaxel compared to one in eight (13 per cent) with mitoxantrone. Docetaxel improved, for example, weight loss, appetite, pain, physical comfort, and bowel and urinary function.[25] Indeed, pain control and quality of life can benefit rapidly, even after the first cycle of chemotherapy (see below).

Combination chemotherapy

Chemotherapies, essentially, poison cancer cells. Scientists developed the first chemotherapies after observing that numbers of white blood cells declined dramatically in people exposed to poison gases used by the military. In December 1942, American researchers used ten doses of one of these poisonous chemicals – nitrogen mustard – to treat a tumour pressing on the windpipe of a 48-year-old silversmith. The tumour, which threatened to suffocate the patient and hadn't responded to radiotherapy, softened and then disappeared. Unfortunately, cancers treated with nitrogen mustard often recur.[12, 26] Doctors still occasionally use nitrogen mustard (now called mechlorethamine, mustine or chlormethine) to treat, for example, certain lymphomas and some leukaemias.

Often the cancer team will combine several drugs, depending on the malignancy, the tumour's stage and your ability to tolerate side effects. In 1957, for example, researchers treated leukaemia with methotrexate or 6-mercaptopurine. Between one in seven and one in five (15–20 per cent) patients entered remission with each drug alone. The combination increased the remission rate to almost one in two (45 per cent).[12] If you have lymphoma, for example, you may discuss combinations with names such as CHOP, VAMP (both combinations of four drugs) and BEACOPP (seven drugs).

The synergistic effect emerges because chemotherapy drugs differ in the way in which they stop cell division, combination treatment 'hitting' the cancer in two or more vulnerable places. Chemotherapy drugs also differ in side effects. So, doctors may be able to combine treatments with side effects that don't overlap allowing a higher total dose of chemotherapy (which maximizes the damage inflicted on the cancer), while limiting side effects and reducing the risk that resistance will develop.

Cycling treatment

You will usually receive chemotherapy over several 'cycles'. You may receive chemotherapy every day for a few days, followed by a 3- or 4-week break. You then have another few days of chemotherapy. Provided you tolerate the side effects, you repeat this cycle several times. During each cycle you may receive the chemotherapy in one or more ways:

- as tablets or capsules you take at home;
- by injection or infusion (using a drip or pump) over a few minutes to several hours in hospital;
- specially trained nurses administer some types of chemotherapy in your home;
- using a small pump that you wear for a week or more.

Chemotherapy's side effects

Chemotherapy drugs don't discriminate between healthy and malignant cells: they have the greatest effect on the most rapidly dividing cells whether or not they are malignant. However, cancer cells generally divide more rapidly than most healthy cells. So, chemotherapy tends to have a greater effect on malignant cells than most healthy cells. Nevertheless, some healthy cells divide rapidly, which contributes to chemotherapy's side effects. The exact pattern depends on the drug. However:

- nausea and vomiting are common partly because chemotherapy damages the rapidly dividing lining of the gut, and partly because the drugs directly affect the part of the brain that tells us we feel sick;
- hair loss follows damage to rapidly dividing cells in the follicles;
- damage to rapidly dividing immature white blood cells increases the risk of infection, so you need to be especially careful about hygiene – such as when preparing food (page 50) – and stay away as much as possible from people with colds and other bugs. Your cancer team might suggest taking antibiotics until white blood cell numbers recover.

As we will see in Chapter 4, you can often help prevent or alleviate many common side effects caused by chemotherapy. Your cancer team will offer you advice tailored to the drugs you're receiving.

You should know what to expect and what to do if the side effect develops, rather than waiting until the problem has become established and more difficult to treat.

Chemotherapy and second cancers

Some cancer drugs – including alkylating agents, such as chlorambucil, cyclophosphamide and melphalan – directly damage DNA. So, some cancer drugs seem to increase the risk of a second primary cancer, which often emerge several years after the treatment of the first malignancy ends.

Chemotherapy can, for example, induce acute myelogenous leukaemia. The risk begins to increase 1–2 years after treatment with alkylating agents, peaks after 5–10 years, and then declines. Unfortunately, these leukaemias often prove difficult to treat. The risk depends on the drug, the combination, the total dose and the duration of therapy.[27]

Radiotherapy

A few months after Röntgen discovered X-rays, Emil Grubbé, a 21-year-old student doctor in Chicago, used radiation to treat an elderly woman whose breast cancer had recurred after a mastectomy. After 18 days', radiotherapy, the cancer shrank. Unfortunately, the malignancy metastasized.[12] Then in 1899, Thor Stenbeck, a doctor in Stockholm, used daily X-ray irradiation to treat basal cell carcinoma (a type of skin cancer) at the tip of a woman's nose. Her treatment lasted three months, but she became the world's first cancer patient cured by radiotherapy.[28]

Unfortunately, X-rays also cause cancer. Indeed, Grubbé had several fingers amputated due to radiation damage and eventually underwent 92 operations to treat the consequences of his early exposure to high doses of X-rays. He died from multiple forms of metastatic cancer.[12, 29] Nevertheless, X-rays revolutionized the diagnosis and treatment of cancer.

Radiotherapy damages cancer cells by shattering DNA and generating free radicals. These free radicals produce breaks in DNA. Many cancer cells are less able to repair this DNA damage than healthy tissues. So, the cancer cell 'self-destructs'. Irradiation also damages the blood vessels that supply the tumour with oxygen and nutrients.

Free radicals

A slice of apple left exposed to the air soon turns brown. Tissue-damaging chemicals called free radicals cause the colour change. Free radicals are waste products produced by many of the normal chemical reactions that keep us alive. Our immune system uses free radicals to help destroy invading bacteria. Free radicals also contribute to the effectiveness of some cancer drugs and radiotherapy.

Free radicals can, however, damage healthy tissue. So, several lines of natural defence protect our cells from free radicals, including a group of chemicals called antioxidants. Unfortunately, pollution, cigarette smoke, pesticides and even sunlight can generate sufficient free radicals to overwhelm these defences. Excessive levels of free radicals seem to increase the risk of developing several serious conditions, including cancers.

Several vitamins, minerals and other antioxidants mop up free radicals, including:

- lutein, found in, for example, green leafy vegetables such as spinach and kale;
- lycopene, the red pigment in tomatoes, apricots, guavas and watermelons;
- vitamins A, C, E and selenium.

Lycopene seems to be especially valuable against prostate cancer. In general, eating a diet rich in antioxidants helps prevent cancer, reduces the risk of a recurrence and boosts your body's innate healing ability. Some antioxidants (such as vitamins C and E, zinc, selenium, and copper) seem to improve healing of surgical wounds, for example.[30] However, because free radicals contribute to the benefits of some chemotherapies and radiotherapy, your cancer team may suggest avoiding large doses of antioxidants (e.g., supplements) during treatment.

Types of radiotherapy

During external beam radiotherapy, the radiographer uses a machine to aim X-rays at the cancer from outside your body. In the early days of radiotherapy, doctors used a single massive dose of radiation, typically lasting an hour. They now use smaller and shorter doses given over several sessions (fractionated radiotherapy), which are just as effective, but much less likely to cause severe side effects. Modern radiotherapy machines also use powerful computers to vary the focus of the beam of radiation to match the tumour's contours. This further reduces damage to the surrounding healthy tissue and delivers a higher dose to the cancer than the older machines.

During brachytherapy, small pieces (called pellets or seeds) of radioactive material are implanted into the tumour, often guided by CT or another imaging technique. The seeds remain in the cancer, destroying the tumour over the next few months as the radioactivity decays to nothing. Another approach uses a thin tube with a tip containing radioactive material. The tube remains in the cancer for several hours or days (depending on the technique) and is then withdrawn. Brachytherapy is most appropriate for small tumours, especially in the prostate, cervix, eye and breast.

Radiotherapy's side effects

Radiotherapy's side effects depend on the dose of radiation, how accurately the technology targets the tumour, and the site of the cancer. In general, however, radiotherapy's side effects include tiredness, weakness, skin reactions and hair loss. The skin reactions, for example, range from a faint redness, to sore itchy skin, to weeping and bleeding. Skin reactions tend to peak during the first two weeks after treatment ends and generally resolve within four weeks.[31]

Radiotherapy can induce second primary cancers, which typically emerge at least a decade after treatment ends, although the risk seems less than with some types of chemotherapy. However, the breasts and the thyroid gland seem to be especially sensitive to radiation. For instance, people with Hodgkin's lymphoma may need high doses of radiotherapy over a relatively large area of their chest, which increases the risk of breast cancer. Women treated for Hodgkin's lymphoma before the age of 30 years seem to be at particularly high risk. The breasts of younger people seem to be especially sensitive to radiation.[27] The benefits, however, generally outweigh the risks. So, have a full discussion with your radiotherapist or cancer team and ask how you can limit side effects' impact.

Hormonal treatments

Hormones are chemical messengers released by glands (such as the pituitary, pineal, thyroid, testicles, ovaries, and pancreas) that control, for example:

- growth and development
- metabolism – the conversion of food into energy
- moods and emotions
- reproduction
- sexual function.

Hormones trigger the growth of certain malignancies in, for instance, the breast, prostate, womb and kidneys. These are *hormone-sensitive* or *hormone-dependent* cancers.

Receptors

Hormones act by binding to specific 'receptors'. Imagine a cell as a car. The receptor is the ignition lock. The hormone is the key. When the key fits into a lock, the engine starts and the car moves. When the hormone binds to the receptor, part of the cell's internal machine starts and the cancer grows. This binding is specific: your key starts only your car. Testosterone doesn't bind to oestrogen receptors, for example. Many of the body's other messengers – such as the transmitters that pass signals between nerves and from nerves to muscle – also act by binding to receptors.

Imagine you have a skeleton key, which fits the ignition lock and switches on the engine. Some drugs act like a skeleton key. The receptor can't distinguish the drug (an agonist) from the messenger produced by the body. Both switch on the cell's machinery. For example, your brain produces natural painkillers called endorphins, which bind to specific receptors. Morphine, commonly used to treat severe cancer-related pain, binds to the same receptors as the endorphins and switches on the same pain-reliving pathways.

Imagine you have another key. It fits the ignition lock, but won't turn. So, the car won't start. But while this key is in the lock, you can't get the right key in. Some drugs bind to the receptor, but don't activate the cell's machinery. These are antagonists or 'blockers'. Tamoxifen prevents oestrogen reaching the receptor, which reduces growth of ER+ breast cancer. Anti-androgens (such as bicalutamide, cyproterone acetate and flutamide) attach to testosterone receptors, stopping the hormone from stimulating prostate cancer (Figure 3).

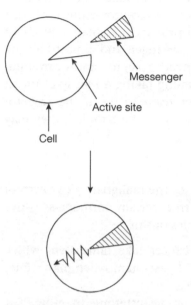

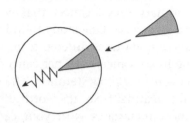

Agonists bind to the active site and
trigger the messages, producing the
same biological effect as the
messenger

The messenger binds to the active
site triggering the messages inside
the cell that produce the biological
effect

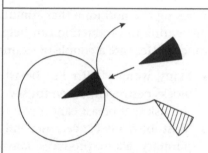

Antagonists bind to the active site and
don't trigger the messages, but they
prevent the messenger from binding,
so blocking the biological effect

Figure 3 Drugs, messengers and receptors

Receptor status

The cancer team can test a sample of the malignancy to see if it
expresses specific proteins (called receptors) for the hormones. For
example, oestrogen and progesterone can stimulate the growth of
some breast cancers. So, the cancer team tests for receptors for these
two hormones and classifies the malignancy as:

- oestrogen receptor positive, ER+ (the abbreviation uses estrogen,
  the spelling in the USA), or negative, ER−;
- progesterone receptor positive, PR+, or negative, PR−.

Doctors call this the cancer's *receptor status*.

As mentioned earlier, cancers can change as they develop. So, a primary breast cancer that is ER⁺ can produce ER⁻ metastases and vice versa. One study found that the receptor status for breast cancer metastases differed from the primary malignancy in about one in six cancers (18 per cent) for oestrogen and almost half (45 per cent) for progesterone.[32] The cancer's receptor status can influence treatment. So, it's worth discussing taking a biopsy of breast cancer metastases with your cancer team to see if the receptor status has changed. (Not all metastases can be sampled: they may be inaccessible, for example.)

Blocking hormones

Blocking the hormone that stimulates the malignancy's growth or preventing its production can help treat certain hormone-sensitive cancers. Here are a couple of examples of this.

- Many women with ER⁺ breast cancer take tamoxifen, which blocks oestrogen. Taken for several years, tamoxifen may reduce the risk that breast cancer will recur.
- Most prostate cancers depend on testosterone to grow. The pituitary gland produces *luteinizing hormone*, which controls production of testosterone by the testicles, and oestrogen and progesterone by the ovaries. Doctors may suggest luteinizing hormone blockers for some prostate and breast cancers.

The choice of hormonal treatment depends on your malignancy and other factors. For example, ovaries stop making oestrogen after the menopause. So, luteinizing hormone blockers work for breast cancer in premenopausal women only. If the cancer no longer responds to a hormonal treatment, doctors describe it as *hormone refractory*.

Side effects of hormone treatments

As you might expect, given the importance of various hormones for our health and well-being, blocking their actions can cause side effects. For example, testosterone increases muscle strength. So, blocking testosterone might trigger fatigue and weakness. Blocking other hormones can induce symptoms, in both sexes, similar to those experienced by many women during the menopause, including:

- hot flushes and sweating: about seven in ten women undergoing hormonal treatment for breast cancer and a similar proportion of men taking some drugs for prostate cancer experience hot flushes;
- memory problems;
- mood swings and depression;
- sexual problems: women may experience vaginal dryness and men may have problems with erections;
- tiredness;
- weight gain.

Other side effects are specific to each hormonal treatment. So, speak to your cancer team and check out the information provided by cancer charities.

Targeted therapies

Targeted therapies (sometimes called biological therapies) influence specific processes that control cancer cells' growth, division, spread and death. Most biological therapies aim to target changes that are unique to, or very much more active in, malignant rather than healthy cells. This limits side effects, although scientists have yet to develop a magic bullet that targets cancer and leaves healthy tissue untouched. Unfortunately, targeted treatments are often expensive, which leads to the high-profile cases where the NHS claims that it cannot afford to fund cancer drugs to gain a few weeks or months of extra life, or to reduce the risk of adverse events associated with conventional therapies.

The mechanism through which these drugs produce their biological effects can be difficult to understand, even for non-specialist healthcare professionals. So, check out the information for patients on charities' websites and don't be afraid to ask questions.

Blocking growth factors

Some targeted therapies – such as trastuzumab and gefitinib – block growth factors. As their name suggests, these messengers tell cancers to grow and spread. For example, receptors called HER2 bind a messenger called *human epidermal growth factor*. Between one in seven and one in four breast cancers express very high numbers of

HER2 receptors (so-called HER2-positive). These tend to grow more quickly than HER2-negative breast cancers. Some gastric (stomach) cancers express high levels of HER2 receptors. Your cancer team will test a sample of tissue to ascertain your HER2 status.

Trastuzumab (also called Herceptin) binds to HER2, which stops the receptor working properly. This interrupts the growth factor's signal. You'll receive trastuzumab only if you are HER2 positive. In about one in seven (13 per cent) of patients, HER2-positive primary breast cancer can produce metastases that are HER2 negative and vice versa[32] – another reason to discuss biopsying secondary tumours.

Blocking blood vessels

Other targeted therapies – including bevacizumab (also called Avastin) – block the formation of the new blood vessels that supply the growing tumour with oxygen and nutrients. Very small tumours can absorb oxygen and nutrients from their surroundings. However, a tumour larger than about one tenth of a millimetre needs its own blood supply.[4] So, the cancer releases chemicals that stimulate the growth of new blood vessels, a process called angiogenesis. Some cancer drugs block the messengers that control angiogenesis, starving the cancer of oxygen and nutrients. Bevacizumab, used to treat a range of cancers, targets a messenger that drives angiogenesis called *vascular endothelial growth factor*.

Targeting genes

Your doctor may test a sample of the cancer to see whether it contains specific mutations. Certain targeted therapies 'switch off' these mutations, usually by blocking an abnormal protein produced by the gene in the pathway that controls cell growth or another critical function, such as removing unwanted proteins. Future treatments may switch particular genes on or off by targeting DNA, although at the time of writing these are experimental.

Immunotherapy

Your immune system protects against invading viruses, bacteria and fungi as well as destroying abnormal, damaged and cancerous cells. Many CAMs seem to stimulate the body's innate healing abilities, including the immune system. Indeed, occasionally the body's innate response is strong enough to lead to the complete or partial disappearance of a malignancy when the patient is not receiving a treatment that could explain the improvement. Doctors call this a *spontaneous remission* (page 97).

Usually, however, the immune system doesn't recognize the cancer as abnormal as 'strongly' as it would, for example, a bacterium. So, the immune response is weaker. Cancers may also produce messengers that dampen the immune response. Drugs called immunotherapies – such as interferons and interleukin 2 – activate the immune system and boost the body's ability to destroy cancer cells. Immunotherapies can, however, overstimulate the immune response more generally producing, for example, flu-like symptoms, rashes or swelling around the injection site, and fatigue.

Vaccinating against cancer

Vaccines protect against serious diseases by enhancing your immune defences. When you are exposed to a virus or bacteria, a vaccine-boosted immune system can usually eradicate the infection before symptoms develop.

Some vaccines prevent cancer. The vaccine against HPV, for example, boosts your defences against this virus, which can cause cervical cancer and some head and neck malignancies. People with chronic hepatitis B virus are up to 100 times more likely to develop hepatocellular carcinoma (the most common liver cancer) than the general population. Indeed, the vaccine against hepatitis B virus was the first immunization that prevented a specific human cancer.[33]

Doctors are beginning to use *therapeutic vaccines* to treat some cancers. In some cases, doctors use samples of the cancer to develop vaccines that stimulate the immune system to attack the tumour. These vaccines will be specific to your cancer – they may not work in another person with the same cancer. Non-individualized vaccines target a specific protein expressed by the cancer but not healthy tissue. Again, the vaccine stimulates the body's white blood cells to attack and destroy the malignancy, but the vaccine would be suitable for anyone who expressed that protein.

At the time of writing, vaccines have shown promising results in melanoma, a type of skin cancer. A variation, which is essentially a modified type of white blood cell, attaches to proteins expressed by the cancer and destroys the malignancy. In a study of people with an aggressive leukaemia known as relapsed/refractory acute lymphoblastic leukaemia, the approach – called CAR-T (chimeric antigen receptor T cells) – eliminated every trace of the cancer in up to nine in ten of those treated. More studies are needed, but therapeutic vaccines and other therapies that boost the immune system are among the most promising new cancer treatments. As it's such a rapidly moving area, it's worth keeping up to date with the latest research, often summarised on patient websites.

Supportive treatments

Depending on your symptoms, general health and well-being, and the type and severity of your side effects, your cancer team may suggest additional 'supportive' treatments.

- Healthy bone marrow makes two million red blood cells every second. Some cancers and treatments can reduce red blood cell production, which may lead to anaemia. *Erythropoietin* increases red blood cell production, which may alleviate tiredness, breathlessness or weakness caused by anaemia.
- Always tell your GP or cancer team if you experience pain – changing your *analgesics* (painkillers) usually helps. Chemotherapy, surgery, radiotherapy and other treatments might shrink or remove some metastases that cause pain.
- Healthy bone marrow normally produces 100 billion white blood cells a day. Some cancer treatments can reduce white blood cell production (so-called leucopenia), leaving you more likely to catch an infection. *Granulocyte colony stimulating factor* (G-CSF) increases levels of white blood cells and so reduces the risk of infections.[4]
- The cancer team may suggest drugs to tackle specific symptoms or side effects, such as nausea, diarrhoea and constipation. Never take any medicine – even one bought without a prescription – without speaking to your cancer team first.

Palliative care

Despite impressive and continuing advances in treatment, there is, unfortunately, little hope of curing most advanced or metastatic cancers. So, your cancer team may offer palliative care. *This does not mean the end of your cancer treatment.* On the contrary, palliative care aims to minimize symptoms, side effects and suffering, while optimizing your quality of life, your ability to reach your goals and make the most of your relationships. Palliative care covers your emotional, spiritual, mental, social and physical, well-being.

Often palliative care will encompass CAMs alongside conventional treatments and may evolve as your needs alter. This means that you and your family need to keep the cancer team up to date with how you feel and any issues you face mentally, emotionally or physically. They'll ask, but don't be afraid to be proactive about discussing your symptoms, needs and problems.

After all, no two people experience advanced cancer in the same way. So, doctors and nurses individualize palliative care to meet your wishes and needs. You can, for instance, decide where you would like to receive care: at home, in hospital or a hospice. This can be flexible: you might consider spending a few days in a hospice to give your carers a break.

Cancer and the carer

Cancer imposes a huge burden on close carers, such as your partner. Family members often endure considerable fear and anxiety, feel sad, helpless and scared, and often report a persistent 'gnawing worry' about the person with cancer.[34] Often they feel that they shouldn't complain or add to your burden. So, they suffer in silence and may not get the help and support they need and that will help them help you.

Indeed, providing care during and after cancer treatment can be the equivalent of a part-time job, taking 20 or more hours a week.[34] Caregivers might need to learn new skills and may experience problems balancing their health needs with those of the person with cancer.[34] After all, cancer is more common as you get older and age increases the risk of numerous diseases. So, carers must make the time to look after themselves and take breaks. A carer taking time out isn't being selfish. They're recharging their batteries, mentally, physically and emotionally, which helps them care for the person with cancer.

The five stages of grief

Grief is a hallmark of the cancer journey. You and your family may experience grief reactions when the doctor told you had cancer, when you learnt the malignancy had progressed and as you approach the end of your life. The psychiatrist Elisabeth Kübler-Ross developed a widely accepted view that suggests that people pass through five stages when they face catastrophic personal loss, such as cancer.

- Denial and isolation – a common initial response. Some people even deny that they have cancer. Obviously, minimizing the impact – so that the cancer doesn't dominate everything – can help you cope. But denial may mean you don't engage with the treatments that could save or prolong your life or save you a lot of suffering.
- Anger – patients ask, 'Why me?' Carers often bear the brunt of this anger.
- Bargaining – patients try to postpone death or ask for a miracle cure for their cancer, perhaps by prayer or a secret pact with God.
- Depression – this can emerge as a 'reaction' to the diagnosis as well as being a side effect of certain treatments.
- Acceptance – the patient reaches peace. Some patients and caregivers find 'meaning' in their illness and use the cancer as an impetus towards spiritual growth.

The order that you move through the stages varies from person to person. You may experience more than one stage at once. You may move between stages. Experiencing these reactions is normal and healthy. But try not to become 'stuck' at any stage.

- Isolation can offer the time and space you need to re-evaluate your life, goals, priorities and problems, and develop a plan to cope with your cancer. However, taken to extremes, isolation encourages apathy and depression. You could become cut off from friends, family, work and other social networks that can offer help and advice.
- Anger can be a valuable safety valve – provided it does not get out of hand. Find time to express your emotions. Counsellors, spiritual advisers and patient groups can help you accept your anger and channel your emotions productively.
- Acceptance may develop into apathy. You need to accept the reality of your situation. But you need to be proactive: stick with your treatment and make plans and set goals to make the most of your life.

Living will

There may come a time when you can no longer easily express your views and wishes about your treatment, your cultural, spiritual or religious practices and beliefs, and food preferences. Perhaps you don't want to upset your family. (For example, some people want to refuse a certain treatment because of the side effects even though they may potentially shorten their life). Perhaps you'll be semi-comatose or too fatigued to summon the energy for a difficult conversation. Perhaps you want to follow particular spiritual or religious practices. Writing a living will (also called an advance statement) helps the cancer team take your views into account even if you can't articulate them.

For example, some people want to stop some drugs, such as painkillers that can cause mental clouding, if they are expected to live only for a few hours. Other people might not want to be kept alive by being fed or given fluids artificially. Some religious and spiritual groups feel that death and dying should be left in God's hands, or believe in religious miracles or redemptive suffering. So, they refuse withholding or withdrawing life support.[35] Your cancer team will respect these wishes and requests, even if they don't hold the same beliefs.

The costs of cancer

Cancer can drain the family's bank account. You will need to pay for transport to hospital and take time off from work, which can cause financial headaches for, in particular, self-employed people. Chemotherapy may mean numerous trips to hospital over several months. You may need new clothing (e.g., if you lose weight or following mastectomy), equipment and modifications to your home. Your family and friends may incur costs, such as losing overtime they rely on.

Speak to your bank or building society, utility companies and so on if you may have difficulty meeting your commitments. You might be able to reschedule loans and mortgage payments. The hospital or a patient group can put you in touch with social workers and helplines to help you access benefits and other support you're entitled to. Budget carefully and look for savings: there are plenty of suggestions on the web and in books.

You decide the contents of the living will, which you can change at any time. But talk your choices through with your cancer team, carers and spiritual advisers. Refusing some treatments in every circumstance could cause you unnecessary suffering and distress. If English isn't your first language, consider asking for an interpreter.

You'll need to ask yourself some tough questions and have difficult conversations with your family and cancer team. Some family members may disagree with your choices, often with the best of intentions. They may be unable to bear the thought of your death. They might want to ensure you receive every possible treatment. They may feel guilty about refusing or withdrawing treatments that may prolong life.[35] A living will can lift some of the burden of decision making from your family's shoulders.

Tips to make taking medicine easier

Before starting a cancer treatment, fully discuss the expected risks and benefits with the doctor or specialist nurse. Even if you don't want to question the team's suggestions, learning about the treatment can help you understand the importance of sticking to their recommendations and how to deal with and prevent side effects.

Think about how the treatment will fit into your lifestyle. You may need to plan childcare, getting lifts to hospital and work around your chemotherapy sessions, for example. So, learn as much as you can about your treatment. You could begin by asking yourself some questions.

- Why is this the best treatment for me at this time in my cancer journey?
- What is the goal of treatment (e.g., are we trying to cure the cancer or tackle a particular symptom?)?
- How and when will I know that treatment is working?
- How and when I know that treatment is not working?
- How will the treatment help me reach my goals?
- What are the risks, complications and side effects? How do these compare to other treatments?
- Will the treatment effect my quality of life for better or worse?
- What can I do to reduce the risk of side effects?
- Will I need to change my lifestyle or activities?

- What should I do if I miss a dose?
- Whom should I contact if I have any concerns or questions?

You and your family will inevitably have questions. But remembering everything you want to ask in the short time you have in the clinic can be difficult. So, keep a notebook or use your smartphone to jot down any questions or anything you don't understand about the cancer and its treatment. Feel free to take notes and ask questions during the clinic visit. Taking a friend or relative with you helps you understand what you discuss during the visit and can refresh your memory.

Remembering to take your treatment

Remembering to take your treatment can be challenging, especially if you need several drugs (including for ailments other than the cancer), you feel depressed and demotivated, or the drugs or cancer affects your memory (see page 36). So, try the following.

- Ask your partner or carer to remind you to take your dose.
- Keep a check list and cross or tick each dose when you take it. You might be able to use an app or another device that tracks your medicine. If you share this either electronically or by pinning the list to the wall, your partner or carer only needs to remind you if you've forgotten.
- Leave yourself notes reminding you to take your treatment on the refrigerator, over your desk, next to the TV, on the bathroom mirror, wherever works for you.
- If you do not have young children or grandchildren you could leave your medicines where they are easily seen, such as on the dining or bedside table or desk.
- Speak to your healthcare team if you have problems opening the packaging or swallowing tablets. There are often ways around the problem. If you have joint pain, for example, a pharmacist can repackage the medicines in containers that are easier to open. Liquid formulations can help if you have problems swallowing. Never open a capsule, crush a tablet or mix a drug with food or drink without speaking to your cancer team or a pharmacist first. You might stop the drug from working or cause side effects.
- Try to take your treatment at the same times each day, which

helps build a routine. You could use an alarm on a watch, phone or timer to remind you.

- Your routine may change when you are on holiday, on a day out, at a birthday or wedding, or away on business. You may need to adjust your timings. Make sure you have sufficient supplies of all your medicines for the time that you are away.

Some people feel that alarms are intrusive and remind them they are ill. If the alarm goes off in public, you might not want to explain about your cancer. You may feel irritated if carers remind you to take a medicine when you already have. So, find what works for you.

Cancer-related cognitive impairment

Some people with cancer experience problems concentrating, focusing or paying attention, which can linger after the initial treatment. Some report memory loss or difficulty remembering names, dates, or phone numbers. Some have problems with comprehension or understanding. Doctors call these and similar problems *cognitive impairment.*

Numerous factors cause or worsen cognitive impairment including some chemotherapies, hormonal therapy, radiotherapy of certain malignancies, stress, chemical changes produced by the cancer and brain tumours. Indeed, up to three in every ten patients experience cancer-related cognitive impairment before treatment. This rises to up to three-quarters during treatment – so-called chemo-brain or chemo-fog. The problem persists for several months after treatment for more than a third (35 per cent) of patients.[36]

Intentionally refusing treatment

These steps can help if the person with cancer unintentionally forgets to take their medication. However, sometimes a person with cancer intentionally doesn't take their medicine as suggested by their cancer team. In one study, about half (55 per cent) taking drugs, including tamoxifen, for breast cancer frequently or occasionally did not take their medicine as recommended. About four in every five (83 per cent) of those who did not take their medicines as suggested said they forgot. But about 1 in 6 (17 per cent) reported that they intentionally did not take their medication.[37]

Some people deliberately didn't take their medication to avoid side effects, such as hot flushes. Other people who deliberately missed their medication viewed themselves as having significantly less influence over their health than patients who followed their cancer team's advice.[37] Perhaps some people feel that not taking a treatment helps re-establish a sense of control. Others may not fully appreciate the benefits of treatment, especially if they experience cancer-related cognitive impairment.

Obviously, a cancer treatment won't work unless you take it. So, if you are deliberately not taking your medicines speak to your cancer team. Ultimately, the choice is up to you. During palliative care, for example, you may refuse a treatment or trade a less effective approach for fewer side effects. Nevertheless, self-help tips and, if necessary, supportive treatments can often manage side effects – so don't suffer in silence. If you feel that you're not in control, try a CAM or counselling instead of ignoring your team's advice.

If you're caring for someone with cancer and you suspect that they are not taking their medicines as suggested, you should gently and non-judgementally raise the issue with the person or the cancer team. You could save or prolong their life.

After treatment ends

Even if you don't need palliative care, managing cancer doesn't end with the last chemotherapy infusion or the final radiotherapy session. You may need to take medicines for several years, perhaps even the rest of your life, to stop the malignancy recurring. You may experience long-term symptoms or problems. You may have to pick up the pieces psychologically after dealing with the diagnosis or the trauma of treatment. So, you'll develop a plan individualized to you that, typically, includes:[2, 38]

- follow up visits with your cancer team;
- changes that help you live with or overcome residual symptoms;
- optimizing general health and lifestyle, including dietary advice to reduce recurrence risk. A personalized dietary and exercise programme can also help rebuild muscle strength, and correct problems such as anaemia or poorly working organs;
- improving your mental and spiritual well-being;
- watching for recurrence and new cancers.

Residual symptoms

Residual symptoms are common among cancer survivors. For example, persistent swallowing problems, dry mouth or poor absorption of nutrients can make eating difficult and lead to, for example, weight and muscle loss.[38] A dietician (ask your GP or a cancer team for a referral) can suggest ways to tackle any nutritional problems.

Fatigue, depression and other mood disturbances, problems sleeping, pain and cognitive issues seem to be particularly common among cancer survivors generally.[34] Indeed, a third of cancer survivors reported that their symptoms were as bad a year after their diagnosis (when they were not receiving treatment) as at the start of their cancer journey.[34] Furthermore, between a fifth and a third of cancer survivors experience fatigue at least five years after their diagnosis or the end of treatment.[34] Some people, for reasons doctors don't fully understand, seem to be especially likely to develop long-term cancer-related fatigue.

In addition, survivors of certain cancers may face specific problems. Urinary, gastrointestinal and sexual problems can persist for years after treatment of pelvic cancers ends, for instance. People who survive breast cancer may endure chronic lymphoedema (page 89).[1]

Sometimes problems arise months or even years after treatment ends, such as osteoporosis following endocrine (hormonal)

Heart failure

Heart failure arises when the heart 'fails' to pump enough blood to meet your body's demands. Doctors divide heart failure into two types.

- In left heart failure, the heart cannot pump enough of the blood that it receives from the lungs. Blood backs up in the lungs (pulmonary oedema), causing breathlessness.
- In right heart failure, the heart cannot pump enough of the blood received from the body. Blood backs up in the legs, ankles, torso and so on, leading to puffiness of the hands, feet or face, discomfort and skin ulcers. This 'congestion' is why doctors often refer to congestive heart failure.

therapies and heart disease after certain types of chemotherapy or radiotherapy. For instance, patients younger than 40 years treated with radiotherapy or chemotherapy for Hodgkin's lymphoma, non-Hodgkin's lymphoma, or testicular cancer are five times more likely than healthy people to develop congestive heart failure, which typically arises more than 10 years after treatment ends.[1]

The long-term psychological burden

Being diagnosed with cancer forces you to confront your mortality, even if the malignancy is not terminal. You might need to adjust your lifestyle or body image (such as following surgery) for the rest of your life. You might need to change or leave employment, especially if you have marked cancer-related fatigue.[34] Not surprisingly, cancer survivors and their families often shoulder a considerable long-term psychological burden.

Fears that the cancer will recur can dominate some survivors' lives after remission. The longer you are cancer free (in remission), the more likely it is that you're cured. For most cancers, the risk of recurrence (relapse) is relatively small after remission has lasted for 5 years. Nevertheless, cancers occasionally recur long after this. About 1 in 200 breast cancers relapse more than 10 years after the initial diagnosis, for example. One woman had a recurrence of her breast cancer 27 years after her initial malignancy.[39]

It is easy to become preoccupied with watching for signs that the cancer is progressing or recurring. Ironically, this increases the likelihood that you'll notice, and worry about, an innocuous symptom. A stomach ache may signal that the cancer has seeded a gastric metastasis. But it's more likely to be indigestion.[40] Anxiety and depression can cause physical symptoms, such as muscle spasms and pain. However, brain metastases, some medicines and uncontrolled pain can cause anxiety and depression. So, while you should be vigilant, try not to worry excessively or become preoccupied. But never ignore a change; always check with your cancer team.

Keeping a note

To help your cancer team better understand your symptoms, you could keep a diary or use a smartphone to note the following.

● How bad was the symptom? Try rating the severity on a scale of

1 (just apparent) to 10 (the worse you have experienced or can imagine).

- If you are nauseous or vomiting, note how many times you are unwell.
- If you suffer diarrhoea or constipation record how many times you pass a bowel movement and the consistency. Ideally follow the Bristol Stool Chart (<www.sthk.nhs.uk/library/documents/stoolchart.pdf>), which is widely used by doctors and nurses.
- What was the symptom? And what did it feel like? Try to be specific. If you experience pain, is it dull and aching? Sharp and stabbing? Or does it feel like electric shocks or pins and needles?
- What was the impact on your life: did the symptoms interfere with your plans, for example, or stop you working or performing a normal activity?
- What you were doing when the symptom occurred? This helps you and the cancer team identify and tackle triggers.
- What, if anything, alleviates the symptom? And how much does it help? Again, you can rate this on a scale of 0 (no effect) to 10 (totally gone).

Collecting such details helps the cancer team understand the symptom's causes and impact, and, in turn, find the best treatment or change in lifestyle. And it helps you stay in control.

Remaining in control

Psychologists refer to your *locus of control*. If you have a strong external locus of control, you feel you have little influence over your life, your health and your cancer journey. You feel that events control you; you do not control events. A strong internal locus of control means you tend to feel that you are in charge of your life, health and cancer journey.

People with a strong internal locus of control are, generally, less likely to be stressed out when facing a life-changing event such as cancer than those with an external locus of control. People with a strong internal locus of control are also more likely to remain motivated about and engaged with treatment and lifestyle changes.

In contrast, if you feel disempowered – that your cancer and its treatment are beyond your control or your life 'is over' – you may be less able to make lifestyle changes needed to cope with treatment or prevent a recurrence. We've seen that people who deliberately didn't take their cancer medicine as suggested by their cancer team often viewed themselves as having significantly less influence over their health than patients who followed the advice.[37]

Such links may help explain why a sense of control seems to improve the prospects for some people with cancer. In one study, women with early breast cancer who felt helpless and hopeless between one and three months after diagnosis were half (53–55 per cent) as likely to survive without showing any signs of the malignancy over the next five to ten years as those who maintained a more positive outlook.[41, 42]

Enhancing your locus of control

Being a passive recipient of health care, just popping the pills or turning up for the chemotherapy session, means control lies 'externally' with your cancer team. In contrast, reading about and trying to understand your cancer and its treatment, tackling side effects and addressing risk factors enhances your internal locus of control. CAMs and counselling can also bolster your internal locus of control. As you address your problems, as you take control of your health, as you reduce your risk factors, you will feel more and more confident. This, in turn, enhances your internal locus of control and boosts your resilience throughout your journey as a cancer survivor.

Setting yourself goals also enhances an internal locus of control. You may need to accept that your cancer means that you can no longer attain a once-treasured ambition, maintain a hobby or develop your career the way you planned. Rather than lament the end of your hopes and dreams, reassess your goals and where you're going. You might need to ask yourself some searching questions about your life and relationships.

- What do you really value? How would you best like to spend your time?
- Make a list of everything you hoped to achieve. What's left? What's still possible (i.e., what could you do in the long term)? What's practical (i.e., what can you do in the short term)? What are the five most important things that you want to do?

- What are your top 20 wishes? Which five of these are the most important?
- Do you keep going over an old argument or an event you regret? Can you resolve the issue, perhaps by building bridges or apologizing?
- Do you want to repair a relationship?
- What do you feel you need to forgive yourself about?
- What upsets you and that you feel is unresolved?

You might find it helps to write these down. You could get out of the house: go to a café or library, for example. The change in environment and fewer distractions can help you focus. If you're worried about anyone seeing your list, use a password-protected file on your computer or phone. You don't have to share this with anyone unless you want to; it's to help you put your thoughts in order. But sharing at least some of your goals with your cancer team may help them adjust treatment to help you meet your ambitions.

Keeping the notes away from prying eyes helps you to be honest, especially when it comes to relationships. You may also need to differentiate between what you *think* you want or need and what you *really* want and need. You may need to ask yourself, honestly, who you are taking the decision for – yourself or someone else. Of course, there are many times in life when you take decisions to meet the needs of other people rather than yourself. However, your true hopes, goals and ambitions can become submerged in other people's expectations and values. You could try to meet other people half way. Then devise a plan and try to take small steps – every day if you can, even if it is a relatively minor advance – that take you closer to your goal.

3

Putting food first

Eating a healthy diet is important for everyone to reduce the risk of cancer and many other diseases. But it's *essential* during all three stages of your cancer journey.

- Keeping your strength up and eating a nutritious diet may reduce the side effects from surgery, radiotherapy and chemotherapy; limit collateral damage; and give your treatment the best chance of working.
- During the recovery phase, a healthy diet helps restore your body's well-being and heals any damage from the treatment or the malignancy.
- During the maintenance phase, a healthy diet may prevent or delay a recurrence, and reduce the risk of, for instance, second primary cancers, heart attacks, osteoporosis and strokes.[3]

Think of your diet as part of your treatment as much as the drugs, surgery or radiotherapy. Indeed, your cancer team's advice may differ to that given for healthy eating generally. For example, in general, everyone should eat a high-fibre diet. But a high-fibre diet could worsen diarrhoea. You also tend to need more energy – and so more calories – than usual during cancer treatment. Some drugs also need you to watch your diet to work effectively: certain foods and drinks may interact with the medicine, for example.

This chapter offers some general advice. There are several cookbooks written specifically for people with cancer. Your cancer team will also offer suggestions tailored to your circumstances and can refer you to a dietician who can help with particular issues and help you make up any nutritional deficit. Oral nutritional supplements, to use the jargon, are now a lot more sophisticated than the milk-based shakes that many GP prescribe by default. The shakes are perfect for some people, but the range of supplements now allows a much more nuanced nutritional approach. A dietician can help find the supplements that are right for you. But food always comes first.

More than nutrition

Animals consume almost anything that their instinct, experience and senses deem edible. In humans, culture and society also determine what food is acceptable and when. Eating guinea pigs, whales and dogs is acceptable in certain parts of the world, but usually inspires revulsion in English-speaking countries. And how often do you eat plum pudding and brandy butter or Brussels sprouts unless it's Christmas? In other words, food is more than a source of energy and nutrients: it has a central place in our culture, society and family life. Even everyday meals are a great way to spend time with your loved ones.

Unfortunately, cancer's impact on eating can place considerable pressure on what should be enjoyable and important social events. Family and friends of people with cancer often regard how much you eat as an indicator of your well-being. They may see weight loss and muscle wastage as a 'harbinger of death'. So, they may pressurize you to eat when you don't feel hungry or to eat more than you feel comfortable. Indeed, family and friends often regard poor appetite as a more serious issue than the person with cancer. Not surprisingly, mealtimes and eating generally can cause conflict and tension.[40]

But try to see the problem from their perspective. The cancer and its treatment can leave your family and friends feeling relatively powerless. They may feel that they can control, at least to a degree, your diet and the amount you eat. If you find that mealtimes are becoming tense, you and your carers could talk to the cancer team or a dietician about diet in general, weight loss and other eating problems. Counselling may help if you feel tense at mealtimes or to help develop strategies that resolve conflicts around diet and the amount you eat.

In addition, as television cookery programmes never tire of reminding us, appearance makes a big difference to how enticing food appears. So, make food look attractive and appetizing, even if you are cooking for yourself. You could, for example, garnish food with parsley, lemon or lime slices, or cherry or sliced tomatoes. Many people with cancer find that they prefer savoury to sweet foods: so you could try adding lemon, lime, chillies and so on to recipes. Cookbooks and the internet offer plenty of other suggestions.

Don't be afraid to ask for help with cooking and food preparation, even if was traditionally your preserve. Fatigue can make preparing food difficult and tiring, for example. Poor nutrition, however, can contribute to fatigue. It is easy to become stuck in a downward spiral.[40] You could make meal preparation part of your 'quality time' with your family. Cooking for a person with cancer helps family and friends show that they care, which is something they may have problems expressing.

Losing weight for cancer survivors

Although patients, professionals and family worry about cachexia and weight loss, some cancer survivors (such as some of those on hormonal treatment) gain weight. Apart from the impact on your health generally, carrying extra weight seems to increase the risk of developing certain malignancies, including kidney, gallbladder, liver, pancreatic and prostate cancer. Indeed, excess body weight caused about 1 in 18 cancers in the UK during 2010.[43] So, there is a risk that excess weight could increase the risk of second primary cancers. If you want to lose weight, it's best to discuss this with the cancer team once your treatment ends and you've recovered.[38]

Anorexia, weight loss, and cachexia

Up to 40 per cent of people with cancer overall and as many as 70 per cent of patients with advanced cancer experience poor appetite and weight loss (anorexia).[44] Cachexia (wasting of fat and muscle), which eventually emerges in up to half of people with cancer, usually develops slowly, beginning with weight loss over several months.[45] Anorexia, weight loss and cachexia undermine people's ability to cope with everyday activities, worsen quality of life, reduce treatment effectiveness and shorten survival.[44, 45]

Factors that can contribute to anorexia, weight loss and cachexia, include the following.

- The site of the tumour can increase the risk of weight loss and cachexia. People with oesophageal, stomach, pancreatic and small cell lung cancers seem to be at especially high risk. Tumours in the oesophagus, for example, can leave you feeling as if food is stuck in the throat. Indeed, four in five patients with stomach or pancreatic cancer, three in five with lung or prostate cancer and one in three of those with breast cancer show marked weight loss over six months.[40, 44, 45]

- Between five and nine in ten of people with advanced cancer report changes in taste and smell, which, if severe, can put people off their food.[40] For example, many people with cancer find they lose their sweet tooth or experience a metallic taste.
- Depression, anxiety, constipation, dry mouth, mucositis (pain and inflammation of the lining of the gastrointestinal tract), nausea and vomiting can make eating difficult.[40]
- Some cancer survivors find swallowing difficult – because of metastases, cancer treatment or medicines for other diseases. For example, some medicines or radiotherapy leave you with a dry mouth.[38]

So, speak to your healthcare team. A combination of managing symptoms and side effects, making changes to your diet, and using oral nutritional supplements usually helps. The following tips may also make life a little easier.

Exercise, yawn and chew well

Light exercise an hour or two before eating can sharpen the appetite:[40] you could walk around the block, for example. Yawning a few times before you start to eat can relax the jaw muscles. Take small mouthfuls and chew the food well.[6]

Graze during the day

Cancer survivors often feel full sooner than when they were healthy. That's one reason why many people with cancer find eating five or six small meals a day easier than having three larger meals. Keep healthy snacks (such as carrot sticks, slices of sweet peppers, and fresh and dried fruits) by you for when you feel peckish.[40] But try to eat one or two of these meals with your family. If you can't finish, and your family is worried, remind them that you are eating more frequently.

Avoid grease and fat

Avoid greasy and fatty foods, especially if you feel nauseous or are vomiting. Eating relatively plain foods – such as rice, pasta, chicken and turkey, bananas, apples, and eggs – can help prevent diarrhoea and nausea. However, adding a knob of butter or stirring in some cream can boost your energy intake without making the food greasy.

Get enough protein

Over the last few years, nutritionists and dieticians have increasingly recognized the importance of ensuring that people who are ill get enough protein. However, many people with cancer fancy only low-protein meals, such as soup and bread for lunch or a bowl of cereal for breakfast. But getting enough protein is especially important for people with cancer.

- Protein helps your body repair damage from the cancer and treatment.
- Protein supports your muscles and help prevent wasting.
- Certain proteins, such as enzymes, have specialized roles that make sure our bodies work properly.
- Protein forms the scaffold that supports the cell. Some cancer treatments kill malignant cells by disrupting this cellular scaffold.
- Protein forms antibodies, which help fight infections.

In general, a healthy diet contains about 50 g of protein a day. Your cancer team will advise what's right for you, which may be more than this: 1 g for each kg of weight for example. However, just eating protein isn't enough. You need to be active to allow your body to make the most of the protein in your diet.

Boosting protein intake

Protein doesn't inevitably mean red meat. Poultry, fish, nuts, eggs, beans and lentils are good sources of protein. Beans and lentils are also high in fibre and help control levels of fats in the blood. You can add lentils to bulk up stews to cut down on meat. Vegetarian cookbooks are full of ideas to help boost your consumption.

Skimmed milk powder is another good source of protein. Dieticians may suggest stirring extra skimmed milk powder into custards, milky drinks and other foods to boost your protein intake. You can also buy protein bars, shakes and fortified foods from health shops. For example, some milkshakes aimed at people who want to lose weight can provide up to 16 g of protein a serving. There's also a range of protein-rich products aimed at the sports market. But remember food comes first. So, use these between meals. And look at your diet. Instead of bread with your soup, try having a chicken or ham sandwich, for example.

Your dietician can prescribe a range of protein-rich oral nutritional supplements, which are an invaluable way of making up any deficit until you can eat a normal diet again. Many people seem to stop taking these supplements after a few days or weeks. But you need to stick with the supplement, just as you would with a medicine. If you don't like the flavour or formulation, there is often an alternative. In addition, dieticians can suggest ways of adding the supplement to normal foods, which helps hide the taste, such as mixing it into a pasta sauce or porridge, and nutrient-rich drinks that you sip during the day.

Limit processed and red meat

The news that the World Health Organization (WHO) considers that there is 'convincing' evidence that eating processed meat causes colorectal cancer captured headlines. The WHO also suggested that red meat 'probably' increases the risk of colorectal and, possibly pancreatic and prostate cancer (<www.who.int/features/qa/cancer-red-meat/en/>). The WHO estimates that:

- each 50 g of processed meat eaten a day increases the risk of colorectal cancer by about a fifth (18 per cent);
- each 100 g of red meat eaten a day increases the risk of colorectal cancer by a similar amount (17 per cent), but further studies need to confirm the link.

Another study reported that each 28 g extra of processed meat a day increased the risk of death from prostate cancer by almost a third (32 per cent), after allowing for other risk factors.[46] Moreover, reducing intake of processed meats would cut the risk of lethal prostate cancer among men over the age of 60 years by just over a tenth (12 per cent).[47] As these examples illustrate, it's sensible to limit the amount of processed and red meat you eat.

Eat fruit and vegetables

Sometimes CAM practitioners and conventional doctors seem to agree on very little. But no-one questions that eating enough fruit and vegetables is the cornerstone of healthy eating. Among the other benefits, a diet rich in fruits and vegetables seems to protect against mouth, throat, oesophageal, stomach, lung and, probably, nasopharyngeal, colorectal, ovarian, womb, pancreatic and liver malignancies.[48]

Tomatoes and prostate cancer

Eating at least seven servings of tomatoes a week seems to reduce the risk of lethal prostate cancer by about a seventh (15 per cent) in men over the age of 60 years.[47] Eating five or more portions a day reduces the risk of death from cancer by a quarter (25 per cent), even after allowing for other risk factors, such as age, smoking, body mass index and alcohol intake.[49]

Tomatoes are rich in a natural pigment called lycopene, which mops up free radicals (page 22). The lycopene in tomato paste, puree and ketchup is easier for the body to use than that in raw fruit, according to the National Cancer institute (NCI). In addition, oils and fats may increase the amount of lycopene absorbed. So, you could toss the tomato salad in olive oil or cook diced tomatoes in olive oil. Not every study suggests that eating tomatoes protects against prostate cancer. But, for men at least, increasing tomato consumption as part of a balanced diet is probably prudent.

Fruit and vegetables are rich in vitamins, minerals, fibre and other nutrients, such as free-radical scavenging pigments. The NHS suggests that most people should eat about 18 g of fibre a day and at least five portions of fruit and vegetables a day. Many scientists now believe that we need to eat at least seven portions a day to gain the maximum overall health benefit. For instance:

- eating between five and seven portions reduces deaths from cardiovascular disease by 20 per cent;
- eating at least seven portions a day reduces the risk of deaths from cardiovascular disease by 31 per cent, after allowing for other risk factors.[49]

How much is a portion?

A portion weighs about 80 g. That's about one medium-sized fruit (banana, apple, pear, orange), a slice of a large fruit (melon, pine-apple, mango) or three heaped tablespoons of vegetables or pulses. This means that, roughly, vegetables and fruits should cover half your plate. Grapefruit and cranberry can, however, interfere with some drugs. So, check before eating these.

Boost your intake by eating a meat-free meal, such as a vegetarian lasagne or stir-fry, a few times each week. Vegetarian cookbooks are

---

Good food hygiene

Several cancer treatments and certain malignancies suppress the immune system, increasing the risk of infection. So, good food hygiene is especially important.[38]

- Be especially careful when handling raw meats, fish, poultry and eggs. If you can, ask someone else to do this step.
- Use one chopping board for raw meat, fish and poultry, and another for vegetables and cooked food.
- Buy pasteurized milk, juices and cheese.
- Thoroughly cook food. Be especially careful with meat, poultry and seafood. Use a thermometer to make sure the meat is cooked through. Eat 'well done', rather than medium or rare, meat.
- Make sure eggs are hard boiled and don't eat food that contains raw eggs. Try not to handle cracked or unrefrigerated eggs.
- Keep food preparation areas and utensils clean, especially following contact with raw meat. Scrub surfaces with hot soapy water.
- Keep raw meats and ready-to-eat foods separate.
- Scrub fruits and vegetables thoroughly, even if you don't eat the skin or peel. Avoid fruits – such as raspberries – that are difficult to wash well. Be especially careful of leafy vegetables, which can hide dirt.
- Store foods promptly at low temperatures and check 'use by' and 'best by' dates.
- Wash your hands thoroughly with soap and water before eating or preparing food.
- When eating out, avoid foods that could become contaminated, such as salads from salad bars, sushi, and raw or undercooked meat, fish, shellfish, poultry, and eggs.

full of ideas, some of which will appeal to even the most ardent carnivore. You could also eat a side salad with each meal and drink smoothies and soups. If you buy juices and smoothies, make sure they are 100 per cent fruit and vegetable, and are pasteurized.

Many CAM diets emphasize eating raw fruit and vegetables. Certainly, cooking can leach nutrients. So, use a small amount of water for the shortest time you can, lightly steam or stir-fry. Wash well, but scrub thoroughly rather than peel potatoes, carrots and so on: the skin is rich in nutrients. You could carry raw carrots, peppers or tomatoes as snacks.

Fibre

During the 1970s, the British research Denis Burkitt noted that colorectal cancer was rare among people in rural Africa who ate a high-fibre diet. Burkitt (who gave his name to Burkitt's lymphoma) suggested that dietary fibre (roughage) reduces the risk of colorectal cancer.[50] Indeed, when researchers combined the results of 25 studies they found that each 10 g daily of dietary fibre reduced the risk of colorectal cancer by 10 per cent. Legumes seemed especially effective: each 10 g reduced the risk by almost two-fifths (38 per cent).[50]

Researchers also increasingly realized that the *Mediterranean diet* (see below) – which is rich in fibre from fruits and vegetables, whole grains, legumes and nuts – protected against certain cancers.[51] A French study, for instance, found that eating more fibre, garlic and onions reduced the risk of breast cancer. Saturated fat intake, however, increased breast cancer risk in post-menopausal women.[52] Meanwhile, UK researchers found that:

- premenopausal women who ate more than 30 g fibre a day were half as likely (52 per cent reduction) to develop breast cancer than those who ate less than 20 g a day;
- cereal fibre accounted for most of the benefit – premenopausal women who ate more than 13 g of cereal fibre a day were two-fifths (41 per cent) less likely to develop breast cancer than those who ate less than 4 g a day;[53]
- fibre did not protect post-menopausal women from breast cancer; however, the other health benefits – such as reduced risks

of heart and circulatory disease, type 2 diabetes and obesity – means that everyone needs to get enough fibre.

How fibre cuts cancer risk

The suggestion that fibre could protect against cancer seems plausible. For example:[50]

- fibre could dilute carcinogens in the gut;
- fibre reduces the time food takes to pass through the gut, so, cancer-causing chemicals have less time to act;
- fibre is rich in antioxidants, vitamins, trace minerals, and other anti-cancer nutrients (whole grains, for instance, are high in folate (vitamin B_9; folic acid) and magnesium, which seem to protect against colorectal cancer);
- high intakes of dietary fibre and whole grains may protect against weight gain, a risk factor for several cancers.

Table 2 Good sources of fibre

Beans: baked beans, kidney beans in chillies and beans in salads	Half a tin of baked beans (200 g) provides about 7 g of fibre
Bran cereal	Make sure it contains at least 6 g of fibre per 100 g
Brown rice	200 g of brown rice contains approximately 1.6 g of fibre
Dried fruit – e.g. apricots	You can carry dried fruit as a snack
Fruit and vegetables	A medium-sized apple provides about 2 g fibre
Jacket potato in skin	A small jacket potato provides about 3 g of fibre
Nuts	Almonds, pecans and walnuts are especially high in fibre
Porridge oats	250 g contains about 2.3 g of fibre
Pulses: beans, chickpeas, lentils; peanuts and peanut butter	80 g of red kidney beans (about 3 tablespoons) contains approximately 5.4 g of fibre, for example
Wholegrain and wholemeal breads, cereals and pastas	Read the packet to see the fibre content

So, get enough of the two main types of fibre.

- Insoluble fibre remains largely intact as it moves through your digestive system, but eases defecation. So, eating insoluble fibre might help if you develop constipation.
- Soluble fibre dissolves in water in the gut, forming a gel that soaks up fats.

A healthy diet contains at least 30 g of fibre a day. Aim to get at least half your starchy carbohydrates from whole grains, such as whole-wheat pasta and bread, and whole oats (see Table 2). You could also try flapjacks and cereal bars. But check with the cancer team about your fibre intake if you develop diarrhoea.

Eat more wholegrains

Grains – the seeds of cereals, such as wheat, rye, barley, oats and rice – have three parts.

- Bran is the outer layer that is rich in fibre and packed with nutrients.
- The germ develops into a new plant and is also rich in nutrients. Wheat germ, for example, contains high levels of vitamin E, vitamin B_9, zinc and magnesium.
- The central area (endosperm) is high in starch, which provides the energy the germ needs to develop into a new plant.

Food manufacturers often remove the bran and germ, leaving the white endosperm. So, whole grains contain up to 75 per cent more nutrients than refined cereals.

Keep your fluids up

It's easy to become dehydrated as you go about your daily life, even if you're not a cancer survivor. In healthy people, the mild dehydration that might arise during daily activities can cause, for example: constipation; poor concentration and memory; increased tension or anxiety; fatigue; and headache.[54, 55] People with cancer face additional problems that make dehydration and these symptoms more likely. You may experience swallowing problems, for example. You may feel too fatigued to get yourself a drink. You may lose fluids because of diarrhoea or vomiting. But it's essential to stay hydrated.

The NHS suggests that adults should drink 1.2 litres (six to eight glasses of water) each day to replace fluids lost in urine, sweat and so on. If you feel thirsty for long periods, you are not drinking enough. You should drink more during exercise, hot weather or when you are in a warm ward or chemotherapy suite. You should also drink more if you feel lightheaded, pass dark-coloured urine or have not urinated in the last six hours. The following tips may help you get enough fluid.

- Carry a water bottle with you and take sips throughout the day. This will help keep you hydrated and, in turn, avoid constipation. Some oral nutritional supplements are sipped between meals, which can help keep you hydrated. Speak to a dietician.
- If you're too fatigued to get up regularly, make sure you keep plenty of bottles of water by your chair or bed.
- Use plenty of gravy, sauces, custards and cream. Keeping food moist can also help you if you have problems swallowing. You can stir extra skimmed milk powder into custards to boost your protein intake.
- Try different drinks – such as Ovaltine, Horlicks, Bovril, milkshakes, cup-a-soups – provided these don't dull your appetite for the meals. These can also boost your intake of protein, energy and other nutrients.
- While you need to drink regularly, try not to consume too much during meals. Fluids can make you feel full up sooner.
- If you have lost fluids from vomiting or diarrhoea, try a drink with electrolytes, such as ones developed for use after a workout. A pharmacist or your healthcare team can also suggest electrolyte drinks.

From the Mediterranean to mushrooms

In the early 1960s, doctors realized that Grecians were surprisingly ancient. In 1961, Grecians' life expectancy at 45 years of age was longer than any other national group then followed by the WHO. Thirty years later, despite a culinary shift to a more typical, less healthy European diet, life expectancy at 45 years of age in Greece (32.5 years) remained second only to Japan (33.3 years) and well ahead of the UK (30.9 years).[56]

The Mediterranean diet probably accounts for much of the Grecians' longevity. Definitions vary between researchers, but typically the Mediterranean diet is rich in fish, fruits and vegetables, whole grains, legumes, nuts, fermented dairy products (e.g., yoghurts and some cheeses) and olive oil. The Mediterranean diet includes moderate amounts of alcohol and limited red meat.[51]

Numerous studies show that the Mediterranean diet is health promoting. For example, during the PREDIMED study, women aged 60 to 80 years ate one of three diets:

- a Mediterranean diet supplemented with extra-virgin olive oil;
- a Mediterranean diet supplemented with mixed nuts;
- a *control* diet of advice to reduce the amount of fat in the diet.[57]

Women who ate the Mediterranean diet with extra-virgin olive oil were seven-tenths (68 per cent) less likely to develop breast cancer than controls. Women who ate the Mediterranean diet with nuts were two-fifths (41 per cent) less likely to develop breast cancer. Olive oil seemed to account for much of the benefit. The authors divided women into five groups based on their olive oil consumption. The women who consumed the most olive oil were four-fifths (82 per cent) less likely to develop breast cancer than those who ate the least.[57] The Mediterranean diet highlights the benefits of a healthy, balanced diet in the fight against cancer.

Green tea and mushrooms

Some cancers are more common in certain parts of the world than others. For example, women from China who eat a traditional diet are four to five times less likely than those from 'industrialized' countries to develop breast cancer.[58] Their traditional diet – which, in many parts of the country, includes green tea and mushrooms – may protect against breast cancer.

In one study, women in China who ate at least 10 g of fresh mushrooms a day were two-thirds (64 per cent) less likely to develop breast cancer than those who didn't eat mushrooms. Those who ate at least 4 g a day of dried mushrooms were half (47 per cent) as likely to develop breast cancer. Drinking green tea boosted mushroom's benefits. Women who brewed at least 1.05 g of green tea dried leaves a day and ate mushrooms were nine-tenths (89 per cent) less likely to develop breast cancer than those who didn't do either. If they ate dried mushrooms and drank green tea, they were four-fifths (82 per cent) less likely to develop breast cancer.[58]

> ### Fungi: neither plant nor animal
>
> Fungi are everywhere from dermatophytes that cause athlete's foot to green growths on stale bread, from black mould at the corners of damp windows to the 1.5 kg white truffle (*Tuber magnatum Pico*) that sold for £165,000 at a 2007 charity auction.
>
> We now know that fungi belong to their own biological *kingdom*. Animals, plants and bacteria each belong to different kingdoms. So, a mushroom in an omelette is as different from the chicken that laid the eggs as it is from the herbs used as seasoning. There are, broadly, three types of fungi. Mould on bread or windows consists of a network of long, fine, intertwined, branching threads, called a mycelium. Some fungi produce *visible fruiting bodies* from the mycelium. These toadstools and mushrooms release spores, the fungal equivalent of seeds. Yeasts, such as those responsible for thrush, are single cells, about the same size as a red blood cell. Some cancer patients are vulnerable to thrush.

Make room for mushrooms

Numerous mushrooms seem to have anti-cancer actions, at least in experimental studies. For example, the snow fungus (sometimes called the silver ear fungus; *Tremella fuciformis Berk*) is widely used in Chinese cuisine and medicine. The snow fungus, among other effects, possesses anti-cancer actions, reduces inflammation and mops up free radicals.[59]

Several species of mushrooms produce polysaccharides (a type of sugar) with potential anti-cancer actions. For instance, polysaccharide K comes from a common mushroom, the Turkey Tail fungus (*Trametes versicolor*; also called *Coriolus versicolor*), which you can see in woods across the UK. (Although never pick fungi unless you are absolutely sure of what you're doing.) Polysaccharide K (also called krestin) is widely used in Japan and some other Asian countries, alongside conventional cancer drugs and radiotherapy, to bolster the immune system's ability to attack the malignancy.[60]

Researchers reviewed 28 studies assessing polysaccharide K in lung cancer, one of the deadliest malignancies. In experimental studies, polysaccharide K boosted the immune system, directly inhibited lung cancer cells, reduced tumour growth and countered the spread of metastasis. In humans, polysaccharide K prolonged survival, improved general well-being (performance status), body weight, fatigue and appetite.[61] Indeed, numerous studies in animals and humans suggest that a variety of polysaccharides from mushrooms reduce side effects from chemo- and radiotherapy.[60]

A wide range of mushrooms is now available from larger supermarkets, which you can add to your meals. Several mushroom-based supplements are available from health shops. If you want to try one speak to your cancer team first. For example, some supplements may interact with other drugs that you are taking.

Green tea

Green tea is another part of the traditional Chinese diet that is rich in chemicals that mop up free radicals. The processing that produces black tea inactivates some of these free-radical scavengers. Oolong tea is chemically between green and black tea.

According to the NCI, some studies suggest that green tea may protect against cardiovascular disease as well as prostate cancer and some other malignancies. One study, for example, enrolled men with high-grade prostate intra-epithelial neoplasia – a precancerous change, analogous to the CIN watched for in cervical cancer screening. About three in ten men with this premalignant change develop prostate cancer over a year. During the study, men took an inactive placebo or three capsules containing green tea catechins (important free-radical scavengers in tea) a day (total 600 mg per day). After 1 year, one man taking the green tea capsules developed prostate cancer, compared to nine taking placebo: a nine-tenths (90 per cent) reduction.[62] Further studies need to confirm the results of this small investigation, but it's promising.

Laboratory studies also suggest that green tea has several anti-cancer actions. Further studies are needed to see how effective green tea is as a treatment for prostate cancer and other malignancies. However, it's worth including in your diet. If you don't initially like green tea, keep trying. You'll soon become accustomed to the taste. You could also, after checking with your cancer team, consider a supplement containing green tea catechins.

Prudent diets and prostate cancer recurrence

In addition to preventing primary cancers, a healthy diet may help reduce the risk that some malignancies will recur. One study, for example, compared two diets eaten by men with prostate cancer:

- a *prudent* pattern: high intake of vegetables, fruits, fish, legumes, and whole grains;
- a Western pattern: high intake of processed and red meats, high-fat dairy and refined grains.

Researchers divided men into four groups, depending on how well they followed the diets.

1 Men who most strongly followed the Western pattern were about 2.5 times more likely to die from prostate cancer over the next 10 years than men who ate the least processed and red meats, high-fat dairy products and refined grains.
2 Men who most strongly followed the Western pattern were two-thirds (67 per cent) more likely to die from any cause, after allowing for other risk factors.
3 Strongly following the prudent diet seemed to reduce mortality by a third (36 per cent).
4 The prudent pattern seemed to protect against deaths from prostate cancer, although further studies need to confirm this finding.[46]

There is a need for further studies assessing the ability of diets to reduce the risk of recurrence. But at the moment, following a healthy 'anti-cancer' diet seems logical, unless your cancer team or dietician makes specific suggestions.

Fish and fish oils

Numerous studies suggest that eating fish helps cut your chance of developing cancer. Fish is a central part of the Mediterranean diet that, as we have seen, seems to protect against breast cancer and some other malignancies. Moreover, eating at least one serving of fatty fish a week seems to reduce the risk of lethal prostate cancer among men over the age of 60 years by almost a fifth (17 per cent).[47]

Fish oil contains about 50 different fats, including the omega-3 polyunsaturated fatty acids (PUFAs), such as eicosapentaenoic acid (EPA) and docosahexaenoic acid (DHA). Among other actions, omega-3 PUFAs:

- reduce blood pressure and improve levels of cholesterol and other fats in your blood, which helps prevent diseases of the heart and blood vessels;
- seem to protect against some common cancers, such as breast, colon and prostate;
- may inhibit transformation of healthy cells into cancers, reduce cell growth, counter angiogenesis and trigger cancer cells to self-destruct;[63]
- optimize the function of platelets, a type of blood cell responsible for forming blood clots (people with thrombocytopenia – which is common among cancer patients, especially those receiving chemotherapy – have low levels of platelets and their blood does not clot properly);
- are important for memory, intellectual performance and keeping joints healthy. Cancer-related cognitive impairment and joint pains are relatively common among people with cancer.

Boosting chemotherapy's benefits

Fish oils may also boost chemotherapy's effectiveness and reduce side effects. For instance, doctors treat some advanced non-small cell lung cancers with the chemotherapy drugs carboplatin combined with either vinorelbine or gemcitabine. Only about three in ten cancers respond and the chemotherapy causes unpleasant side effects affecting, for example, the gut, blood and heart.[64, 65]

Adding an average of about 2 g EPA and 0.3 g DHA a day to these drugs more than doubled the proportion of cancers that shrank compared to chemotherapy alone (60 per cent versus 26 per cent). Fish oil users were also about twice as likely as those treated with chemotherapy alone (80 per cent and 42 per cent respectively) to show cancers that shrank or remained stable. In part, these benefits probably reflect the greater proportion of people using fish oil who completed chemotherapy (87 per cent and 57 per cent). After a year, three in five (60 per cent) of those who'd taken fish oils were still alive compared to about two in five (39 per cent) of those who received chemotherapy alone.[64, 65]

Adding fish oil did not worsen chemotherapy's side effects. Indeed:

- people receiving chemotherapy alone lost, on average, 2.3 kg. People receiving fish oils maintained their weight;
- seven in ten (69 per cent) patients taking fish oil gained or maintained muscle mass;
- three in ten (29 per cent) patients treated with chemotherapy alone maintained muscle mass and, on average, this group lost 1 kg of muscle.[64, 65]

Choosing fish

Humans can make omega-3 fatty acids from another fat in green leafy vegetables, nuts, seeds and their oils. But it is a slow process. So, in general, try to eat at least two portions of oily fish per week (a portion is about 140 g once cooked). If you are eating canned fish, check the label to make sure processing has not depleted the omega-3 oils. If at first you do not like the taste of oily fish, do not give up without trying some different sources and a few recipes (see Table 3). There are plenty of suggestions on the internet and in cookbooks. If you still can't boost your intake, discuss a supplement with your cancer team.

Table 3 Examples of fish and seafood high in omega-3 fatty acids

Anchovy
Black cod (sablefish)
Crab
Dogfish (rock salmon)
Halibut
Herring
Mackerel
Mussels
Oysters
Pilchards
Rainbow trout
Sardines
Salmon
Tuna (especially bluefin)

Adapted from the University of Michigan and the British Dietetic Association

Supplements

Cancer survivors need to tread carefully with supplements. Several studies, for example, suggest that high doses of some vitamins can reduce the risk that certain cancers may recur. However, further studies need to determine the size of the effect and who benefits. Until these questions are resolved, it's best to avoid very high doses of any vitamin and mineral unless your cancer team agrees.

Indeed, high doses of certain vitamins, minerals and other supplements can cause side effects or interfere with conventional cancer treatments. For example, cells need folic acid (vitamin B_9) to make DNA. Some chemotherapy drugs, such as methotrexate, kill cancers by interfering with the way the cell uses folic acid.[38] So, adding folic acid could undermine the effectiveness of chemotherapy regimens that include methotrexate. Check with your cancer team before taking a supplement and ask if there are any dietary restrictions. For instance, some foods (such as certain breakfast cereals, and yeast and beef extracts) are fortified with folic acid.

Some vitamins, such as vitamins C and E, are powerful antioxidants, mopping up free radicals. However, some cancer drugs and radiotherapy work, at least in part, by generating free radicals that damage cancer cells. So, in theory at least, antioxidant vitamins might undermine the effectiveness of some cancer treatments. Other researchers think that antioxidants could help protect normal cells from collateral damage.[38] Again, it's prudent to avoid high doses of antioxidant supplements and ask your cancer team if you are unsure. Nevertheless, vitamin supplements may help with some specific problems as the following examples show. If you want to try these, check with your cancer team.

Vitamin E

Vitamin E might alleviate the nerve damage caused by certain cancer drugs, including the taxanes, such as paclitaxel. This nerve damage can cause unpleasant symptoms including loss of feeling, 'pins and needles' and pain (a condition called *peripheral sensory neuropathy*). Supplements containing vitamin E, glutamine (an amino acid, one of the building blocks of protein), and a naturally occurring chemical called acetyl-L-carnitine seem to reduce the risk of developing, and the severity of, peripheral sensory neuropathy caused by taxanes.[66] Vitamin E might also alleriate menopausal symptoms and stomatitis (page 87).

Several foods are rich in vitamin E, such as seeds, nuts, oily fish and wheat germ. Plant oils (e.g., soya, corn and olive oil) are also especially rich in vitamin E. Unfortunately, processing often removes vitamin E from plant oils. So, buy cold-pressed plant oils.

Vitamin D

Vitamin D is essential for, among other actions, making sure we absorb sufficient calcium and phosphorus from our diet. We need calcium and phosphorus for healthy bones and strong teeth.[67] Calcium is also involved in muscle contractions (including our heartbeat) and ensuring that blood clots normally. Phosphorous also, for example, helps the body use carbohydrates and fats, make protein and store energy. Vitamin D roughly doubles the amount of calcium absorbed (from 10–15 per cent to 30–40 per cent) and boosts uptake of phosphorus (from 60 per cent to 80 per cent). However, most cancer patients are deficient in this vital vitamin.[68]

In 1980, American researchers suggested a link between cancer and vitamin D, after noting that deaths from colon cancer rose the further you got from the equator and in areas with less sunlight. Since then, studies have confirmed that vitamin D seems to reduce the risk of developing several malignancies, including breast, lung and bladder cancer.[132]

Sunlight, which triggers the skin to make vitamin D, is the main source of this essential nutrient in the UK. However, from around mid October to the beginning of April, sunlight in the UK does not include the wavelength needed to make vitamin D.[67] In addition, your cancer team might suggest using a sunscreen to help protect your skin. Sun protection factor (SPF) 15 sunscreens can reduce the amount of vitamin D you make by 99 per cent.[68]

The recommended intake for adults is 400 International Units (IU) – equivalent to 10 micrograms – of vitamin D a day. Oily fish, eggs, and fortified fat spreads and breakfast cereals contain vitamin D: 85 g of cooked salmon contains about 566 IU.[69] A large egg yolk contains approximately 41 IU of vitamin D.[67, 69]

A fifth of UK adults and up to a third of children aged 4 to 10 years have low vitamin D levels. So, discuss a supplement with your cancer team. You can also protect your bones with exercise, and by avoiding smoking and excessive amounts of alcohol.[44] Your doctor may also suggest certain drugs to boost your skeleton's strength.

Restrictive diets

Some CAM practitioners suggest restrictive diets or even fasting to treat cancer. The idea is, essentially, that fasting deprives the cancer of the nutrients it needs to grow and survive. Some CAM practitioners also believe that fasting helps the body get rid of toxins, some of which, they suggest, are carcinogenic.

It sounds logical – and in the past some conventional researchers and doctors advocated severely restricting nutritional intake to treat cancer. We now know, however, that fasting starves your healthy tissues and may shorten survival, undermine your quality of life, exacerbate fatigue, and delay and lengthen recovery.[38] If anything, you'll need to eat more calories, protein and other nutrients to maintain your weight and aid your recovery.[38] So, it's best to avoid restrictive diets and fasting.

Juicing is a great way to get enough fruits and vegetables. Juice therapies take this a step further and use fresh fruit and vegetable juices as the main source of nourishment. Some CAM practitioners suggest that juicing stimulates the immune system, lowers blood pressure and aids detoxification. While you need to get enough fruits and vegetables, most dieticians and doctors would suggest juices only as part of a balanced diet. Furthermore, a juice diet can cause or exacerbate diarrhoea.[44] The foundation of well-being – whether or not you have cancer – is a healthy, balanced diet that's right for you.

4

Tips to help specific issues facing survivors

This chapter looks at some lifestyle changes and other tips that may help prevent or manage particular problems you might face at some time during your cancer journey. Given the wide range of cancers, symptoms, side effects and treatments, these are only principles. Any advice that your cancer team offers overrides these suggestions. If you feel unwell at any time, contact your GP or cancer team.

Nausea and vomiting

Between a tenth and a quarter of people receiving chemotherapy endure persistent nausea and vomiting.[70] At least seven in every ten people with advanced cancer report chronic nausea.[40] Certain drugs – cisplatin, for example – seem to be especially likely to cause vomiting.[12] Some cancers cause nausea and vomiting, by, for example, affecting the gastrointestinal tract or changing the blood's chemistry.

Nausea and vomiting evolved to protect us: you expel hazardous material before it can do you harm. Indeed, nausea and vomiting are among our body's strongest and most basic reactions. Even the thought or a reminder (*cues*) of the chemotherapy triggers the reaction – so-called anticipatory nausea and vomiting. Doxorubicin, for instance, is a red-coloured infusion that commonly causes nausea and vomiting. Some patients experience nausea and vomiting when they see the colour red outside the chemotherapy suite. Moreover, if you expect that you'll experience nausea and vomiting when you receive chemotherapy, the more likely the symptoms are to occur.[70]

Your doctor can prescribe drugs called anti-emetics, which reduce the frequency and severity of nausea and vomiting. The following may also help.[5, 70, 71]

- Many people find that hypnosis counters anticipatory nausea and vomiting.

- Avoid fatty, greasy and fried foods. Eat small amounts of plain foods when you feel able. Try baked, boiled or mashed potatoes rather than chips; or turkey or chicken instead of red meat. You could try poached egg on dry toast or a chicken breast with plain noodles or rice.
- Grape juice may reduce the frequency and duration of nausea and vomiting.
- If the smell of cooking triggers nausea, eat cold meals or prepared foods.
- Dry foods, such as toast and crackers, may help settle a sensitive stomach.
- For centuries, traditional healers have used ginger to alleviate nausea from a variety of causes. Some people find that ginger alleviates chemotherapy-related nausea and vomiting more effectively than some anti-emetics. So, try crystallized ginger, ginger tea or ginger biscuits.
- Vomiting can lead rapidly to dehydration. So, sip plenty of fizzy drinks (such as ginger beer, mineral water, lemonade or soda water) slowly through a straw. If you find a straw difficult to use, try a bottle with a sports cap.
- Rinse your mouth before and after meals, which helps get rid of any lingering tastes.
- Sit up or lie back with your head raised for at least an hour after eating.
- Relaxation techniques can help reduce nausea and vomiting before eating.
- Counselling can help break any psychological link between anticipatory cues or certain foods and nausea and vomiting.

Constipation

Numerous factors can trigger constipation in people with cancer, including some painkillers, dehydration and certain malignancies. So, if you think you have constipation, keep a diary using the Bristol Stool Chart (page 40) for a few days and see your doctor. But don't take laxatives unless your healthcare team tells you to.

Dehydration can make stools harder. So, drinking between six and eight glasses of water a day can help. Some people find that not drinking alcohol, coffee, tea and grapefruit juices, which can make you urinate more, helps avoid dehydration. Bland foods – such as rice, banana and apples – and eating more fibre may also help avoid constipation.

Take regular exercise, ideally for at least 30 minutes a day. And try to have regular bowel movements. You might find defecating after breakfast easier, when the bowel's contractions tend to be strongest. Try to go the toilet at the same time each day.

Diarrhoea

Diarrhoea has numerous causes other than cancer and its treatment, including infections, irritable bowel disease, laxative overuse and reducing the dose of, or stopping, some painkillers. So, if you think you have diarrhoea, keep a check using the Bristol Stool Chart (page 40). If you have four or more episodes a day, see your doctor as soon as you can.

Sometimes a doctor may prescribe (or advise you to buy) anti-diarrhoeal drugs. In some case, they'll suggest you keep this at home and start taking the drug at the first sign of diarrhoea. However, never buy a treatment for diarrhoea (or any other problem) without speaking to your cancer team first: some anti-diarrhoeal drugs could cause additional problems or interact with other elements of your treatment.

The following tips may help alleviate diarrhoea.[44, 66, 71]

- Avoid caffeine, alcohol, fruit juices and smoothies, high-fibre, fatty, greasy and spicy foods. Try eating plain food (such as bananas, white bread, white fish, chicken or turkey) in small, frequent meals.
- Eat foods rich in pectin, which is the natural gelling agent found in ripe fruit used to make jams and jellies. Eating less fibre and more pectin-rich foods helps build your stools' consistency (Table 4).
- Diarrhoea can mean that you can lose large amounts of potassium, a mineral which, for instance, nerves and muscles need to work properly. As a result, this can leave you feeling weak and fatigued. So, eat foods high in potassium (Table 4).
- If you experience diarrhoea, drink at least 2–3 litres a day. Diarrhoea can lead rapidly to dehydration.

- Probiotics help restore the natural balance of bacteria in your gut, which can become disrupted by cancer and its treatment as well as by supportive care, such as antibiotics. Changes to the balance of bacteria in the gut can trigger diarrhoea. Ask your cancer team or dietician if you are not sure which probiotic is right for you.
- Try eating foods at room temperature: cold and hot foods tend to stimulate the gut.

Good hygiene is very important if you develop diarrhoea. Clean yourself carefully after each bowel movement. Use soft wipes and pat rather than rub. You can apply a barrier cream to protect the delicate area around the anus.

Table 4 Foods rich in pectin, potassium or both

Foods rich in pectin	Foods rich in potassium
Apple: peeled or as sauce, without spices	Apricot nectar
Asparagus tips	Asparagus tips
Avocados	Avocados
Bananas	Bananas
Beets	Fish
Plain pasta	Peach nectar
Potatoes: baked, without skin	Potatoes: boiled or mashed, without skin
White bread	
White rice	

Fatigue

Fatigue is one of the most common, disabling and distressing problems experienced by people with cancer. People with cancer-related fatigue feel that they have no energy. They feel tired all the time, and physically, emotionally and mentally exhausted. Rest and sleep don't alleviate their profound tiredness. Their body, especially their arms and legs, may feel heavy. They may experience problems concentrating or find that they can't think clearly. Indeed, some people with severe cancer-related fatigue may be unable to perform everyday activities, such as eating, shopping, working, exercising or even personal hygiene.[2]

At least four-fifths (80 per cent) of cancer patients experience fatigue during treatment with chemo- or radiotherapy and most (60–90 per cent) regard fatigue as their most disabling symptom.[40] Occasionally, fatigue is so profound that patients discontinue treatments, contemplate suicide or wish for an early death.[40] So, how can you reduce fatigue's impact?

Causes of cancer-related fatigue

Numerous factors potentially cause or contribute to cancer-related fatigue, such as: [2, 34, 40, 44]

- surgery, chemo- and radiotherapy;
- disrupted sleep, anaemia, infections and poor nutrition;
- cognitive problems, depression and pain;
- some cancers release chemical messengers that undermine your energy (when chemo- and radiotherapy destroy or damage the cancer, the tumour may release a flood of chemicals into the blood that trigger anxiety, sleep problems and fatigue).

Cognitive problems, depression and pain can cause or contribute to cancer-related fatigue. In addition, fatigue can increase the likelihood of cognitive problems, depression and pain. Depression, for example, can sap your motivation and energy. However, doctors sometimes inappropriately blame psychological factors when their suggestions fail to alleviate cancer-related fatigue.

Keeping a diary helps you and your cancer team identify the causes of fatigue. The diary also helps assess fatigue's impact on your ability to perform the normal activities of daily living and on your quality of life. Understanding the triggers and consequences helps identify the best way to help you. Your diary should record: [5]

- how bad the fatigue feels: try ranking severity on a scale of '0' for no fatigue or tiredness to '10' for the worst fatigue you've experienced or can imagine;
- how much the fatigue interferes with your daily life; you could rank this from '0' for no interference to '10' for being unable to get out of bed or out of a chair;

- your sleep patterns: this helps reveal any link between your fatigue and poor sleep hygiene or poorly controlled pain;
- your daily activities: this helps identify any triggers;
- what you have tried to address the fatigue and any improvement. You could rate the effectiveness on a scale of '0' for no improvement to '10' if the fatigue resolved.

Dealing with cancer-related fatigue

Unlike nausea, vomiting and pain, doctors have few drugs that can help people with cancer-related fatigue, unless anaemia, an infection or depression contributes.[44] Fatigue often improves after the cancer treatment ends and tends to be worse early in the journey. It seems as people learn to live with the cancer, they know what to expect (the severity of cancer-related fatigue sometimes comes a shock) and what helps.

Planning, prioritizing and pacing

Planning, prioritizing and pacing allow you to spend your time and energy on activities you value most. So, list things that *you have to do* and what you can leave or ask someone else to do. And make a list of who you can ask for help, for what and when (so that, for example, it fits into their commitments).

Family and friends are usually more than willing to help, but often don't know what to do or feel uncomfortable asking. They could help by, for example, giving you a lift to hospital, looking after children, cooking or doing the housework. Often your family and friends will feel better because they can do something to help.[6, 40, 44, 71]

Plan your daily routine, which should include regular rest and relaxation. You may find that you need to add extra periods of rest before or after activity or visitors. Take a break if you feel you need to rest even if it's unscheduled. Struggling on just makes matters worse. Nevertheless, you need to strike the right balance between rest and activity. Excessive rest can sap your energy and interfere with sleep.[6, 40] Your diary can help you discover the balance that's right for you.

Find time to exercise and other tips

Although you may feel that you are too tired to work out, exercise is one of the best ways to counter cancer-related fatigue. Exercise can prevent fatigue from getting worse, even in people with advanced cancers,[40] and brings a wide range of other health benefits, from stronger bones, to sharpened appetite to stress reduction. So, include exercise in your plans.

Several other tips may help you live with cancer-related fatigue.[6, 40, 44, 71]

- A motorized scooter may help preserve your independence.
- You could ask your cancer team or GP to refer you to an occupational therapist, who could suggest changes around the house that help conserve energy, such as grab rails, raising toilet seats or putting chairs near stairs.
- Overuse of painkillers, sedatives and some other drugs can cause or contribute to fatigue. If you suspect that a treatment might be contributing to your fatigue, speak to your cancer team. There is usually an alternative.
- Some people find that fatigue undermines memory and concentration. So, try making notes, keep lists and try to stick to a routine.
- Try to distract yourself. Watch a DVD, read or listen to music or a podcast – anything that takes your mind off the cancer and your fatigue.

Fatigue among carers

Carers often endure profound tiredness and marked sleep disturbances. After all, caring for someone with cancer can be mentally, physically and emotionally exhausting. So, carers:

- might need to prioritize the demands on their time and plan accordingly;
- could learn some stress and time management techniques;
- should try to get enough rest and relaxation, and take part in activities that they enjoy at least a couple of times a week;
- should discuss respite care with the cancer team. Recharging your batteries will help you better care for the cancer survivor.

- Try to take part in activities you enjoy several times a week.
- Try yoga, mindfulness, meditation, guided imagery and progressive muscle relaxation (see Chapter 5).
- Think about your diet. Cells use a sugar called glucose as fuel. Digestion breaks complex carbohydrates and simple sugars into glucose. Blood glucose levels shoot up within a few minutes of swallowing a sugary drink. Converting starchy carbohydrates into sugars takes longer. So, you might find that eating, for instance, rice, chapattis, yam, noodles, cereals, pasta, potatoes and bread maintains your energy levels better than simple sugars.

Sleep disturbances

Between a quarter and two-fifths of survivors experience sleep problems. Indeed, many survivors find that disrupted sleep is the most severe long-term symptom and the impact may be more pronounced than the side effects of the cancer treatment. Caregivers can experience sleep disturbances that are as marked as those endured by the survivor.[34] Some studies also link sleep deprivation – for example among shift workers – with an increased risk of breast and prostate cancer.

Not surprisingly, sleep disturbances and fatigue are closely related. In one study, two-thirds (68 per cent) of survivors with fatigue experienced sleep disturbances, compared to about a quarter (28 per cent) of survivors without fatigue.[34] Sleep problems arise:[40]

- as a cancer symptom;
- as a side effect;
- from poorly controlled pain or nausea;
- following disruptions to your routine due to care;
- from stress, depression or anxiety.

Many of these can affect the sleep of carers as well as the survivor. But your cancer team will often by able to help, perhaps by adjusting your treatment. So, don't suffer in silence.

People with cancer and their carers should also follow the good sleep hygiene tips in Table 5. If you cannot sleep, get up and do something else. Watch the TV or read – nothing too stimulating – until you feel tired. Lying there worrying about not sleeping keeps you awake.

Table 5 The principles of good sleep hygiene

- Exercising just before bed can disrupt sleep, although regular exercise aids sleep and helps counter cancer-related fatigue
- Try to avoid naps. If you experience cancer-related fatigue, you should schedule rest regularly throughout the day
- Avoid alcohol. A nightcap can help you fall asleep. However, as blood levels fall sleep becomes more fragmented and lighter. So, you may wake repeatedly in the latter part of the night
- Avoid stimulants, such as caffeine and nicotine, for several hours before bed. Try hot milk or milky drinks instead
- You need to remain hydrated. But do not drink too much fluid (even non-alcoholic) just before bed as this can mean regular trips to the bathroom
- Do not eat a heavy meal before bedtime
- Go to bed at the same time each night and set your alarm for the same time each morning, even at the weekends. This helps re-establish a regular sleep pattern
- Make the bed and bedroom as comfortable as possible. Invest in a comfortable mattress, with enough bedclothes, and make sure the room is not too hot, too cold or too bright
- Do not worry about anything you have forgotten to do. Get up and jot it down (keep a notepad by the bed if you find you do this a lot). This should help you forget about the problem until the morning
- Try not to take your troubles to bed with you. Brooding makes problems seem worse, exacerbates stress, keeps you awake and, because you are tired in the morning, means you are less able to deal with your difficulties. Try to avoid heavy conversations and arguments before bed
- Use the bed for sex and sleep only. Do not work or watch TV

Pain

Pain is often cancer's most feared symptom. Certainly, pain potentially undermines almost every aspect of your life, from your day-to-day mood, to your will to live, to your relationships and social life, to your ability to sleep, exercise and eat.[40] Pain is a biological alarm that evolved to warn you that something's wrong: that's why it can be so hard to ignore. Chronic pain can seem like a loud alarm that you just can't turn off.

Pain can have numerous causes, including the tumour, its

treatments and the aftermath of an operation. Some diagnostic procedures can be uncomfortable or even painful. For example:

- nurses administer many cancer treatments by infusion, which can cause pain, swelling and skin reactions around where the tube enters your vein;
- severe mucositis (see page 86) can be very uncomfortable;
- some cancer drugs can cause pain in the joints and muscles;
- radiotherapy can cause sore and even painful skin reactions.

Unfortunately, pain does not always subside after treatment ends. About two-fifths of long-term survivors of breast cancer experience chronic pain, for example. Similarly, a study that included people with a variety of cancers found that a fifth reported pain at least two years after diagnosis.[34]

Don't grin and bear pain

Modern painkillers (analgesics) and other treatments can almost always adequately control cancer-related pain. So, make sure that your cancer team knows when and where the pain develops, and its severity. They'll also need to know the type of pain – you could keep a diary (page 39). A dull pain may have different causes and treatment from pins and needles, for example, even if they are equally unpleasant. So, tell your cancer team if:[44]

- you experience pain in a different part of the body from usual;
- the pain is getting worse or the painkillers don't seem to work as well as they did;
- you experience numbness, weakness and tingling;
- you lose sensation in part of your body;
- you experience changes in your ability to control your bladder or bowels;
- the pain interferes with your daily life.

Your doctor will probably begin by trying to control your pain using 'simple' painkillers, such as aspirin and paracetamol. If these prove inadequate, they may try mild opioids (such as codeine). Finally, they can offer strong opioids, such as morphine. You are extremely unlikely to become addicted if you follow the cancer team's advice, who can reassure you if you're worried about dependence. Follow your healthcare team's advice, but as a rule, take painkillers at regular intervals (such as every 3 to 6 hours) or as the pain begins to emerge. 'Grinning and bearing' the pain means that analgesics typically take longer to work.

Sometimes an operation or radiotherapy can alleviate pain. For example, surgery or radiotherapy might remove or shrink a tumour that presses on a nerve. Surgeons can also cut certain nerves that carry the pain signal. Many people find hypnosis, acupuncture and massage help control pain.

Peripheral neuropathy

Some drugs and certain malignancies may damage nerves, which can lead to a problem called peripheral neuropathy, characterized by, for example:

- numbing, tingling or loss of feeling in the limbs;
- feeling as if you are wearing a sock or glove;
- burning, stabbing or electric-like pains;
- being very sensitive to touch.

If you develop any of these symptoms, tell your cancer team: analgesics and some other drugs may help. Avoiding alcohol and, as far as possible, repetitive activities that may stress nerves (such as golf, tennis, playing an instrument or using a computer keyboard), biofeedback, acupuncture, hypnosis and relaxation techniques (see Chapter 5) may also help.[44]

Muscle and joint pain

Some chemotherapies – including taxanes and vinca alkaloids – and certain cancers can cause painful joints (arthralgia) and muscles (myalgia). Often simple painkillers help. Try the following.[44]

- Applying a heating pad, hot water bottle, an ice pack or a packet of frozen peas to the painful joint or muscle.
- Soaking in a warm bath. Try some aromatherapy or use Epsom salts in the water, which some people find eases sore muscles and joints. Always check with your cancer team first: some aromatherapy essences may not be suitable and you need to make sure that anything you add to your bath won't undermine your skin care.
- Try massage, acupuncture, hypnosis and relaxation techniques.

Anxiety and pain

Doctors may suggest drugs or counselling (page 101) to help reduce anxiety and depression, which commonly exacerbate pain. In one study of women with metastatic breast cancer, mood disturbances and believing that pain suggested the cancer had progressed increased pain severity.[40] In another study, three-fifths of cancer patients feared that pain meant their cancer was getting worse. These people were more likely to report anxiety and depression than those who did not consider pain to herald a deterioration.[40]

It's almost as if anxiety, depression and fears of progression turned the 'pain volume' up. Yet pain severity does not always reflect the extent of the underlying tissue damage and does not inevitably indicate that the cancer has worsened. So, discuss your concerns with the cancer team. Several CAMs can help by directly treating the pain or by reducing anxiety and depression. We'll return to the ways you can tackle mood disturbances later in this chapter.

Caring for your skin, nails and hair

Skin, nails and hair divide rapidly. You replace about 30,000 skin cells every minute, for instance.[8] So, cancer and its treatment can take its toll on your skin, nails and hair.

Some cancer drugs may cause an area of dry, scaly skin. Some might trigger an itchy, red area. Some might cause pus-filled pimples that look like acne. Radiotherapy can mean that your skin blisters and peels, leaving moist red areas.[6] Your cancer team can suggest steroids, antibiotics and other drugs that may help protect and heal your skin and dressings that should speed the healing of any damage following radiotherapy.[6] So, mention any change in your skin to your cancer team.

Protecting your skin

You can take several steps to protect your skin.[6]

- If you develop a skin problem or have received radiotherapy, check which creams, cosmetics, medicines, tapes and plasters, and bath products you can use.
- Don't use perfumed soap, skin-care products, cosmetics or deodorants.

- Use a moisturizer regularly on dry skin. Check with the cancer team or radiotherapist which is the best one to use.
- Avoid long, hot showers and baths. Wash in warm or tepid water and don't stay in too long. Pat yourself dry with a clean, smooth towel. Don't rub.
- Make sure the house isn't too warm and try a humidifier if the air seems dry.
- Avoid wool and synthetic fibres. Wear loose-fitting, soft cotton clothes.
- Avoid wet shaving. Don't use hair-removing creams or wax, especially in the area being treated.
- Wash sheets and clothing in mild detergents.
- You can take up swimming after you check with the cancer team. However, chlorine can dry skin, so use a moisturizer.
- If you develop diarrhoea, be particularly careful about personal hygiene: chemicals in faeces can damage the delicate skin around the anus.

Protection against the sun

Safe sun practices prevent most skin cancers. But you need to remain vigilant even if you have already had a skin cancer. For example:[72]

- three-fifths (60 per cent) of people with their first non-melanoma skin cancer develop another of these malignancies within 10 years;
- if it isn't their first, a similar proportion (62 per cent) develop another non-melanoma skin cancer within 2 years;
- nine in ten (91 per cent) develop another non-melanoma skin cancer within a decade.

So, keep an eye open for any changes to your skin. Examine your skin every month: a check only takes 10 minutes or so. Take a selfie, use mirrors or ask a friend or family members to look at 'difficult to view' skin areas. Marking the location of each mole, birthmark, bump, sore, scaly patch, and so on, on an outline of the body (<www.skincancer.org/skin-cancer-information/early-detection/body-map>) helps identify changes.

Your cancer team will tell you what to watch for. However, if you are unsure check and tell your GP or cancer team if you see:

- any lesion (e.g., a spot, blemish or mole) that is growing, bleeding, changing in appearance, or never heals completely;
- a discoloured red, scaly patch on the skin that may itch;
- an irregularly shaped new mole, or an existing mole that changes shape.

Safe sun tips

Radiotherapy and some other cancer treatments can leave your skin highly sensitive to sun – so-called photosensitivity reactions. In other words, you are much more likely to get sunburnt than you were before treatment. Sometimes the skin may be so sensitive that you get sunburnt indoors (through windows) or on cloudy days.[6] This may mean that you may have to use sun cream on cloudy days and during the winter.

Apply sun cream with a sun protection factor (SPF) of 15 or more at least every two hours. Some people will need a minimum SPF of 30 and ideally 50, either because of the malignancy (e.g., in those with skin cancers) or its treatment (e.g., drugs that cause photosensitivity reactions). Ask your cancer team for advice about the right SPF for you.

The sun cream should protect you from both UVA and UVB. Ask your pharmacist if you are unsure. Apply the sun cream more frequently if you are sweating or swimming. Cover as much skin as possible, including your ears and bald patches or where you've lost hair and use a lip balm. In addition:

- wear a broad-brimmed hat, UV-protective sunglasses and clothing with a close weave and that covers as much skin as possible;
- wear UV-protective swim and beach wear;
- avoid direct sunlight as much as possible, especially between 11 a.m. and 3 p.m.;
- if you are particularly photosensitive, use window films that block UVA and UVB in the home, office and car;
- avoid sunbeds or sunlamps.

Tackling itch

Once again, cancer-related itch has several causes. For example, a cancer can release chemicals that triggers itch. Often the irritation subsides if treatment shrinks the cancer. In other cases, your bile duct can become blocked by a tumour. The build-up of bilirubin and other toxins can cause itch. Surgeons may be able to unblock a blocked bile duct or prescribe a drug called cholestyramine, which binds itch-promoting bile salts.

Your cancer team may suggest anti-histamines. These block the action of histamine, a chemical messenger that triggers itch. Some anti-depressants may be especially helpful if peripheral neuropathy or other forms of nerve irritation cause the itch. Doctors can also prescribe steroids as creams or tablets. These dampen the activity of cells that trigger itch. Contact your cancer team if:

- the itching worsens or becomes more widespread;
- an itchy area on your skin becomes more red and sore, leaks pus or smells;
- you can't sleep because of the itch;
- the treatments don't seem to be working.

Self-help tips for itch

The following tips may help you deal with itch.

- Several CAMS – including acupuncture, hypnosis or relaxation therapy – can help.
- Apply a cold pack or a packet of frozen peas to the itchy area. Some people find that rubbing, tapping, pressing the itchy area or gently pinching the skin nearby helps.
- Apply an unscented and colourless moisturizer after bathing or when the itching is uncomfortable: ask your cancer team or pharmacist which is the best one to use.
- Don't take too many baths and don't spend longer than about 20 minutes in the bath, use lukewarm water and little or no soap. You can use an emollient suggested by your doctor, pharmacist or nurse instead of soap.
- Some people find oatmeal baths help.
- Pat skin dry with a towel rather than rubbing with a towel. But dry yourself well to help reducing chafing and the risk of fungal infections.
- Drink 2–3 litres of fluid a day: dehydration can trigger or exacerbate itch.
- Keep rooms cool and humid. Hot and dry atmospheres can make the itch worse.

- Keeping your nails short and wearing soft cotton mittens and socks helps avoid skin damage if you can't help scratching.
- Avoid things that might make your itch worse, such as certain hair and cleaning products, scented products or preparations containing lanolin.
- Wearing loose-fitting cotton clothes often helps: wool and man-made fabrics can irritate the skin.
- Try to take your mind off the itch by watching TV, listening to music, reading – or whatever distracts you.

Nail problems

We spend millions each year on manicures, false nails and polishes to make our nails attractive. Nails also protect your fingertips and, by supporting the other side of the finger, help you make precise delicate movements and enhance the sensitivity of your touch.

Some cancer treatments can leave nails brittle or affect the nail bed. So, watch for any changes, such as separation of the nail from the nail bed, discolouration or an increase in milk spots. The following may also help:

- use a moisturizer regularly;
- wear gloves, which helps protect delicate nails;
- avoid false nails;
- keep your nails short, but don't push back the cuticle, which can increase the risk of infections, or have aggressive manicures or pedicures;
- don't bite your nails;
- keep your hands and feet as dry as possible.

In general, nail problems resolve when treatment ends. But see your cancer team if the nail problems are painful or mean you are less able to perform your normal activities.

Hair loss

Hair loss (alopecia) is, perhaps, the most familiar side effect of cancer treatment. Healthy head hair grows by approximately 12 cm (5 inches) a year and you normally lose about 100 hairs a day. As we've seen, chemo- and radiotherapy target rapidly dividing cells. So, losing a few more hairs is common. But don't worry if you see a few extra hairs on the brush. You need to lose at least half your hair before anyone else will notice.[44]

Hair loss typically begins 2–3 weeks after chemo- or radiotherapy starts, usually beginning on the crown and above the ears. In addition to scalp hair, chemotherapy can mean you lose beard, eyebrows and pubic and body hair. Unless you received very high levels of radiotherapy, hair normally grows back within 3–5 months of the end of treatment – although it may be a different texture or colour. Sometimes regrowth begins before treatment ends.[44]

Speak to your healthcare team, a counsellor or a patient support group if your hair loss causes you distress. The following may help limit the impact.

- Cut your hair short when you start treatment; any loss may seem less dramatic and you regain your style quicker.
- Hair loss can leave skin sensitive or tender, even before the loss becomes visible. So, be careful when you shave, depilate or cut your hair.
- Massaging the scalp removes dry skin and flakes.
- Do not wash your hair every day. Use mild or baby shampoo.
- Don't scrub your hair dry vigorously. Pat your hair dry gently.
- Brush your hair gently using a soft hairbrush, especially when it begins to regrow. Limit pinning, curling, or blow-drying with high heat.
- Avoid using chemicals (e.g., hair colour) until your hair has regrown. Test any chemical on a small patch of hair first. Avoid hair colour for at least three months after your treatment ends.
- Choose a soft, comfortable covering for the bed pillow.
- Think about a wig or hairpiece. A hairdresser can help you style the wig or hairpiece, which you should have fitted properly to stop scalp irritation.

Depression and anxiety

Is it any wonder that a person whose partner dies from cancer becomes depressed? Is it any wonder that a person with cancer feels depressed about their loss of bodily function or surgery has left them disfigured? Is it any wonder that they feel anxious about being a burden to their families or friends, about the cancer recurring or financial problems caused by the disease?

That so many people with cancer *do not* develop profound depression or anxiety amazes me. Some people even manage to use cancer as a springboard to personal growth. Nevertheless, depression is common among people with cancer, even if they survive the initial malignancy. About two-fifths of long-term survivors of breast cancer experience depression, for example,[34] which can dramatically undermine their quality of life.

In addition, brain tumours or metastases can cause psychiatric symptoms, such as depression, mania, hallucinations, anxiety disorders or anorexia nervosa. Indeed, depression might be the only sign of a brain tumour.[73] That's another reason for survivors to get new or worsening depression checked.

More than low mood

Depression is much more debilitating, intrusive and distressing than a low mood or 'simple' sadness that's natural when you face a life-transforming event, such as cancer. Depression is a profound, debilitating mental and physical lethargy, which is why it can make fatigue worse. Depression is a pervasive sense of worthlessness, despite evidence to the contrary. Depression is an intense, deep, unshakable, guilt and crushing sadness. As William Styron remarks in *Darkness Visible*, depression 'remains nearly incomprehensible to those who have not experienced it in its extreme mode'.

The symptoms of depression differ from person to person. Nevertheless, doctors recognize several core symptoms. For example, people with depression typically spend a considerable time ruminating about the past. They feel guilty about mistakes, when they let others down, and events and acts that they regard as immoral or sinful. Some patients and carers may develop depression because they regard the cancer as 'punishment' for their sins.

When to see your doctor

The more symptoms in Table 6 (overleaf) you have, the more likely you are to have depression, especially if they persist and interfere with your day-to-day life. So, see your GP as soon as you can if you have little interest or take little pleasure in doing things you used to enjoy, or you feel down, depressed or hopeless for most of the day, every day, for more than two weeks. See your doctor *urgently* if you experience any of the following:

Table 6 Examples of depression's core symptoms

Examples of psychological symptoms of depression

Considering suicide, self-harm, or taking steps towards suicide

Continuous low mood or sadness

Feeling anxious or worried

Feeling hopeless and helpless

Feeling irritable and intolerant of others

Feeling ridden with guilt – especially if the guilt is excessive or unjustified

Feeling tearful or crying

Lack of interest in things or activities – especially if these were once important or enjoyable

Lacking motivation

Low self-esteem

Procrastination – finding it difficult to make decisions

Examples of physical symptoms of depression

Change in appetite or weight (usually decreased, but may increase)

Changes to the menstrual cycle

Constipation

Feeling lethargic – moving more slowly than usual

Lack of energy

Loss of libido

Sleep disturbances – such as finding it hard to fall asleep at night (more than about half an hour) or early-morning waking

Speaking more slowly or less than usual

Unexplained aches and pains

Examples of social symptoms of depression

Avoiding contact with friends and family

Avoiding social activities

Neglecting and not being interested in your hobbies and interests

Poor performance at work (e.g. poor concentration, lack of motivation and absenteeism)

Problems in your home and family life

Adapted from NHS Choices

- you feel that life is unbearable;
- you are considering or taking steps towards suicide or self-harming;
- you can't meet your work, social and family obligations or lack the motivation to work towards your goals, exercise or follow the treatment or fatigue plan;
- you hear voices in your head – which are usually critical or defamatory – or experience visual hallucinations. Hallucinations can be symptoms of a very serious condition called psychotic depression. In addition, some brain cancers and certain medicines can trigger hallucinations.

If you feel suicidal or are getting to the end of your tether then see your GP, go to Accident & Emergency, speak to the cancer team or phone a helpline such as:

- Samaritans on 08457 90 90 90;
- Breathing Space on 0800 83 85 87;
- HOPELineUK on 0800 068 41 41.

Physical symptoms of depression

Depression affects the body, mind and emotions. For example, about two-thirds of people with depression develop physical (also called somatic) symptoms, such as:[74, 75, 76]

- aches and pains;
- back pain, especially in the lower back;
- breathing difficulty or breathlessness;
- chest pains;
- digestive problems – nausea, diarrhoea or constipation – and stomach pain;
- dizziness, light-headedness or feeling faint;
- headaches;
- problems swallowing;
- tiredness, exhaustion and fatigue.

These overlap with many symptoms of cancer or side effects of certain treatments. Once again, keeping a diary may help distinguish symptoms of depression. For example, the aches and pains that arise as a somatic symptom often seem to be 'everywhere' rather than affecting a specific part of the body, such as muscles or joints. Even so, get unpleasant, painful or limiting symptoms checked.

Anxiety

Anxiety evolved to produce physical, mental and behavioural changes that warn us of, and help us deal with, potential dangers, such as walking alone late at night or dealing with a serious disease. Anxiety disorders arise when our natural 'fear' reaction is out of proportion to the threat, is excessively prolonged or interferes with our everyday life.

Essentially, people with anxiety are highly sensitive to potential threats. Their enhanced fear response leaves them *hyperaroused*. Those with anxiety may feel restless, panicky, on edge and irritable. They may feel that their heart is racing or palpitating. They may have difficulty concentrating and sleeping. They may feel sweaty, dizzy, need to urinate a lot and suffer chest and abdominal pain.[44] People with anxiety usually recognize that their concern is excessive.

Answering yes to either of the following questions suggests that you might have anxiety.[77]

- During the past four weeks, have you been bothered by feeling worried, tense or anxious most of the time?
- Are you frequently tense, irritable and having trouble sleeping?

Anxiety's physical symptoms

Anxiety increases mental alertness and heightens your senses to help you detect danger. Adrenaline and other chemicals flood your body. So, your heart beat increases. You breathe more rapidly. You sweat. Blood flows from your skin and your intestines to your muscles. That's why we go pale when stressed or frightened. Muscles surrounding the hair follicles tighten. That's why we get goose bumps. Our pupils dilate: we're wide-eyed with fear.

This flood of chemicals can cause physical symptoms: we're 'sick with fear', have 'the runs' or complain of 'butterflies in the tummy'. Anxiety also causes symptoms – such as tense sore muscles, 'pins and needles' and shortness of breath – that overlap with those caused by some cancers and certain side effects. So keep a note about when and where the symptoms arise.

Post-traumatic stress disorder

About a third (35 per cent) of cancer survivors have post-traumatic shock disorder (PTSD) – the condition closely related to anxiety that also causes the shell shock endured by the military. Almost nine in ten (86 per cent) people with cancer experience some PTSD symptoms, but don't cross the threshold for the full-blown condition.[78]

People with PTSD often report flashbacks 'out of the blue' and vivid dreams and nightmares about the trauma, such as when they were told they had cancer or it had recurred, pain from the malignancy or its treatment, or long stays in hospital. They typically avoid places and people that evoke memories of the cancer, refuse to speak about their experiences and feel constantly on guard or emotionally numb. PTSD can place a considerable strain on relationships, and increases the risk of suicide, drug and alcohol abuse, and aggression.

Treating anxiety and depression

You should begin by trying to identify why you feel anxious or depressed. Try to be specific rather than just saying 'the cancer'. What particularly bothers you? Fear of death? Concerns over pain? Worries about recurrence? The impact on your family? Ask yourself what unanswered questions and unresolved issues you have about the cancer and its treatment: both commonly cause stress and anxiety. Ask your cancer team or a charity for the answers.

Try to avoid becoming preoccupied by symptoms and watching for signs of recurrence, another common cause of anxiety among cancer survivors. A stomach ache may still be indigestion even if you have cancer. Indeed, anxiety can cause muscular aches and pains, which you may worry are signs of recurrence. While carers need to watch for new signs and symptoms, asking too regularly can fuel this preoccupation.

If anxiety, PTSD or depression interferes with your daily life, speak to your GP or cancer team. They can address particular problems that evoke anxiety, such as poorly controlled pain. They might also suggest anti-depressants and anxiolytics. These don't cure depression or anxiety in the way that, for example, antibiotics cure bacterial infections. However, anti-depressants and anxiolytics may alleviate symptoms, offering you the chance to address the causes. Talking treatments, such as CBT and counselling (page 101), often address thoughts and behaviours that trigger depression, anxiety or PTSD. In addition, numerous CAMs mentioned in Chapter 5 relieve anxiety and depression including: relaxation, guided imagery, massage, music and art therapy, and yoga.

Ask yourself what and who helped you get through difficult times in the past. Who and what made matters worse? You can draw on these resources and insights, which are often more extensive than you realize, to ease you along your cancer journey. Try to take part in more family and recreational activities, which can help take your mind off your problems. Try to get out and about in nature, which seems to have an anti-anxiety action in addition to the benefits of exercise alone (page 120). And cut back on caffeine and alcohol, both of which can worsen anxiety. Drinking excessive amounts of alcohol can also exacerbate depression.

Mucositis and stomatitis

Up to two in every five people undergoing chemotherapy and up to half of those receiving both chemotherapy and radiotherapy develop mucositis: pain and inflammation of the soft layer of tissue lining the gastrointestinal tract from the mouth to the anus. Stomatitis refers to mucositis in the mouth. Indeed, mucositis and stomatitis are almost inevitable with chemotherapy and radio-therapy for cancers of the head and neck and are very common after bone marrow transplants.[6, 44]

In general, mucositis emerges about a week after the start of radiotherapy and usually lasts for 2–3 weeks after treatment ends. Mucositis and stomatitis may leave you susceptible to oral thrush (oral candidiasis), which causes white patches on the mouth and tongue.[6, 44]

Symptoms of mucositis and stomatitis

Speak to your cancer team if you develop any of these symptoms, which could suggest mucositis:

- dry, cracked lips
- pain (for example, in the throat, lips and mouth)
- difficulties swallowing
- ulcers and sores on the mouth and tongue
- bleeding (from the gums or mouth, for example).

> ### Bleeding gums
>
> Some cancers and cancer treatments can affect platelets, the blood cells responsible for clots. So, contact your cancer team if you feel you bleed excessively when you brush or floss. You could ask for a check-up from a dentist before you start cancer treatment. This can help address any problems that could get worse during treatment.[6]

Tackling mucositis and stomatitis

Poor oral hygiene and badly fitting dentures can exacerbate mucositis and stomatitis. Take the following steps.[6, 44, 66, 71]

- Gently brush and floss at least twice a day unless your doctor tells you otherwise. Use a soft (or a child's) toothbrush. You might find that a toothpaste for sensitive teeth is more comfortable than your usual brand.
- Rinse your mouth out with warm salt water or a non-alcoholic, unsweetened mouthwash after each meal and at bedtime. If you want to rinse more often, check which mouthwash to use and how often you should use it with your cancer team or dentist. You should avoid mouthwashes containing alcohol, for example. In addition, your cancer team or dentist may be able to suggest painkilling mouthwashes.
- A vitamin E supplement and 'swish and swallow' formulations of glutamine may reduce the frequency, severity and duration of oral mucositis. Tablets and other oral formulations of glutamine do not seem to be as effective as 'swish and swallow'. Ask your cancer team about these and other antiseptic and anti-inflammatory mouthwashes, gels, etc. Your pharmacist or cancer team can suggest treatments for mouth ulcers and sores.
- Vaseline or a lip balm may ease sore lips.
- Sucking ice cubes or flavoured ice pops can alleviate pain.
- Avoid spicy, salty or acidic foods, and raw vegetables, granola, toast and other 'rough' foods. If hot and warm foods irritate your mouth, eat cold foods or meals at room temperature.
- Try eating soft food, such as mashed potatoes, scrambled eggs, macaroni cheese, cottage cheese, soft fruits or purees, soups, milk and yoghurt shakes.

- If you want to drink alcohol, avoid neat spirits.
- Some people find that tomato, grapefruit and some orange juices irritate their mouths. Drink plenty of water, if necessary using a straw or a bottle with a sports cap.

Dry mouth

Dry mouth (xerostomia) can lead to, for example:

- difficulty speaking, eating or swallowing;
- halitosis (bad breath);
- recurrent mouth infections, including thrush;
- taste changes;
- tooth decay and gum disease.

Radiotherapy can, for instance, damage your salivary glands. In general, your salivary glands will start working properly 3–4 months after the end of radiotherapy. However, if you received a large dose of radiation, dry mouth may last longer or even be permanent.[6] Several cancers, certain drugs – including some anti-depressants, anti-histamines and diuretics (water tablets) – and dehydration can reduce saliva production.

Tips to tackle dry mouth

The following tips may help.[6]

- Chew sugar-free gums, sweets or pastilles.
- Cook with plenty of sauces and gravy.
- Avoid dry foods – such as crackers, flaky pastry and chocolate – which can stick to the lining of the mouth.
- Regularly sip cold water or unsweetened drinks. Some people find that fizzy drinks are better for a dry mouth than still drinks.
- Rinse your mouth out with a teaspoon of baking soda (sodium bicarbonate) dissolved in a glass of warm water.
- Smear your mouth and tongue with olive oil or melted butter, which some people find especially helpful at night.
- Cut out smoking and alcohol and, for some people, tea and coffee, which can dry the mouth. Avoid mouth washes containing alcohol.
- Suck ice cubes and lollies.
- Suck pineapple chunks.

- Your cancer team or local pharmacist could suggest artificial saliva, which comes as a spray, gel or lozenge. You can use these before and during meals.
- Your cancer team or GP can prescribe a drug called pilocarpine, which may stimulate glands damaged by radiotherapy to produce more saliva.

Lymphoedema

In some people with cancer, damage to, or removal of, parts of the lymphatic system (page 6) can lead to local fluid retention and tissue swelling. This problem, called lymphoedema, usually causes swelling in the limbs. Sometimes, however, swelling can extend to the groin, face, neck and genitals. Lymphoedema can impair body image, sexuality, social activities and your ability to perform some jobs or activities around the house.[44] If you develop lymphoedema, the following may help.[44]

- Many people find strengthening and aerobic exercise especially helpful. But avoid heavy lifting (more than about 7 kg or 15 lbs) or vigorous repetitive motions against resistance.
- Be careful to avoid injuring parts of the body affected by lymphoedema.
- Ensure good hygiene to avoid infections. Watch for any signs of an infection – such as a raised temperature. Speak to your GP or cancer team if you think that you may have developed an infection.
- Avoid keeping your legs still for a long period, such as during air travel.
- Try to keep at a healthy weight.
- Eat a low-salt, high-fibre diet, which helps remove excess fluids.

Pyrexia

Some cancers and certain treatments can increase the chance that a survivor will catch a viral, fungal or bacterial infection. Pyrexia – a high temperature – is part of the body's natural response to infections. In addition, some tumours produce chemicals that cause fever.

Pyrexia usually passes as your body adjusts – a bit like resetting the thermostat on your central heating. In the meantime, drugs such as paracetamol, ibuprofen or aspirin can help bring your temperature down and alleviate pain and discomfort. You may need to take doses every 4 to 6 hours until your temperature returns to normal. Ask your cancer team which drug is best for you. You should not take aspirin, for example, if you have a low count of platelets or are at risk of bleeding for other reasons. In addition:

- remove excess clothing and bed linen;
- have tepid baths, showers or sponge down;
- drink lots of cold fluids;
- suck on ice cubes or ice lollies;
- open the window or have a fan in the room;
- rest.

If you have the chills, change wet bed linen and clothes. Stay away from draughts and keep windows closed. Avoid the temptation to huddle up under a blanket. Your temperature is still high and you will just make the fever worse or last longer.

Contact your GP or cancer team urgently if you:

- feel very unwell or your temperature is very high (for example, over 39.4°C; 103°F);
- your temperature doesn't return to normal after a couple of days;
- you feel faint and lightheaded, which might be a sign your blood pressure is low;
- you feel confused or very agitated;
- you feel very drowsy.

Menopausal symptoms

Some drugs and hormonal treatments can cause 'menopausal' symptoms, including:[44]

- forgetfulness and poor concentration;
- hot flushes;
- mood changes;
- night sweats;
- sleep disturbances;
- urinary incontinence;

- vaginal dryness;
- changes to the pattern of, or the end of, periods.

Four-fifths of women aged less than 25 years of age recover their normal menstrual cycles after chemotherapy ends. Women over the age of 40 years are at higher risk of permanent menopause.

Men taking hormonal treatments, such as for prostate cancer, can develop some 'menopausal' symptoms, including hot flushes, sweating and breast tenderness. Doctors can prescribe drugs that can alleviate some of these symptoms. You could also try:

- a low-fat diet, which may reduce the severity and frequency of menopausal symptoms;[44]
- avoiding spicy foods, caffeine and excessive amounts of alcohol, which may reduce hot flushes;
- vitamin E might reduce the number of hot flushes triggered by hormonal treatment;[2]
- relaxation, acupuncture, quitting smoking, maintaining a healthy weight and regular exercise may reduce the severity and frequency of menopausal symptoms.[44]

Sexual problems

Sexual problems and worries about sexual performance associated with cancer and its treatment can cause considerable stress and affect relationships. Indeed, between 20 per cent and 100 per cent of cancer survivors report some degree of sexual dysfunction. But this depends on the site of the cancer. At least half of those with breast, prostate, colorectal and gynaecological cancers endure long-term sexual problems, for instance.[44] Despite being common, many people suffer in silence rather than seek the help that's readily available.

You should, for example, ask about any impact on sexuality or fertility when deciding on treatment. If appropriate, ask about sperm banking or egg storage.[44] And check when it's safe to have penetrative sex, especially if you have brachytherapy, surgery or radiotherapy to your pelvis.[6] In addition, radiotherapy to the pelvis can cause bands of scars (called adhesions) that narrow or shorten the vagina. If you are having radiotherapy to the vagina, you can use a vaginal dilator – which is shaped like a tampon – to stretch the vagina, prevent adhesions and break up scar tissue. Regular sex also helps.[6]

Give your sex life a boost

The following might help give your sex life a boost.[44]

- Fatigue can mean you feel too worn out to have sex. So, try the tips on page 67.
- Avoid large meals if you think you're likely to have sex. Digestion diverts blood from other parts of your body, including from your sexual organs, to your gut.
- Change position – the other partner being on top can help prevent breathlessness or relieve the pressure on sore parts of the body.
- Non-irritating lubricants (ask your pharmacist or cancer team) can help if you experience vaginal dryness.
- Living with stress, anxiety, depression and altered body image can affect desire and libido. If you get an erection during the night or in the morning, the cause may be more psychological than physiological. Relaxation, anti-stress techniques and advice from a counsellor or a patient group often help if stress undermines your sex drive.
- Doctors can prescribe several drugs that help impotence. But never buy any drug over the net. If you want to try a herbal treatment for impotence check with your cancer team first to ensure that it does not interact with your cancer treatment.
- Several drugs that lower blood pressure, certain treatments for depression and anxiety, and some other medicines can cause impotence. If you think that a drug might be causing or contributing to your problems, speak to your doctor. There is usually an alternative.
- Avoid anything that triggers nausea, which may include perfumes, aftershaves, scented candles and so on. A light snack before you expect to have sex could settle your stomach.
- Pain can make sex difficult. Take analgesics an hour before if you expect to have sex, try different positions and support painful areas with cushions or pillows.

Partners of people with cancer can also help.

- Spend time with your partner or go on 'dates'. Some carers find that the increased opportunity to be intimate when looking after a survivor increases sexual desire. Consider making time with your partner a *priority* when planning to cope with fatigue.
- Reassure your partner that you love them and find them attractive despite any physical changes or side effects.
- Discuss with your partner any fears or concerns you have about being intimate. If necessary, swallow your embarrassment and speak to the healthcare team, a patient support group or a counsellor. They can reassure you if, for example, you are worried that being intimate might cause the cancer survivor pain.
- Be patient. It might take a few weeks for a person to get their sexual confidence back. Talk to your healthcare team, a counsellor or a patient support group if you feel these approaches are not making a difference.
- Keep an open mind. You might have to find new ways to make love, such as being more forward, becoming the 'dominant' partner or using sex toys and lubricants. Sexual pleasure is not always about penetration, it's also about intimacy.

5
CAMs can help

Many patients and carers find that CAMs help ease the heavy spiritual, emotional and psychological burden imposed by cancer. CAMs can help control symptoms, improve well-being, enhance quality of life, bolster a healthy lifestyle and augment the efficacy of conventional treatments. *However, never stop a treatment or reduce a drug's dose without speaking to your cancer team first. And never believe practitioners who claim to cure cancer.*

The examples in this chapter illustrate some of the CAMs that in clinical studies helped certain people with cancer. Unfortunately, there is only space to skim the surface of this vast area. As is always the case in cancer, there are, however, no guarantees. You will invest time, energy, emotion – and often money – in some CAMs. Yet the cancer may still progress or return. Nevertheless, CAMs help make the cancer journey easier for many people.

Types of CAMs

You can choose from numerous CAMs from acupuncture to zootherapy – using animals as a treatment. Broadly, however, CAMs fall into five groups.[7]

- *Biologically based therapies*, such as diets, vitamins, herbalism and aromatherapy.
- *Energy fields*; some CAM therapists believe that energy fields surround and penetrate the body. They believe that they can manipulate these energy fields using, for example, traditional acupuncture, Reiki and reflexology.
- *Manipulative and body-based CAMs*, such as chiropractic, osteopathy, shiatsu, massage and the Alexander technique depend on manipulating or moving parts of the body.
- *Hypnotherapy, visualization and spiritual healing*, for example, are used to enhance the mind's ability to influence the body. Some

approaches – such as counselling – are predominately psycho-logical. Nevertheless, by addressing the psychological burden imposed by cancer, patients often feel better physically.

- *Complete systems*, which include homeopathy, Ayurveda and Traditional Chinese Medicine (TCM).

Some CAMs fit into more than one group. During shiatsu, healers apply rhythmic pressure to parts of the body that, they believe, are important for the flow of the 'life force' or qi. So, shiatsu is a manipulative and an energy field therapy. In addition, healers often take elements from more than one approach to meet their clients' individual needs. Naturopathy combines diet with, for example, herbalism, acupuncture and counselling.[7]

A blurred boundary

It's sometimes hard to see the boundary between mainstream therapy and CAMs. Ayurvedic medicine is mainstream in India, but a CAM in the UK.[7] It's also sometimes hard to see the boundary between alternative and complementary therapies. Broadly, however, alternative therapies *replace* conventional treatments. Sometimes the patient's intent makes the difference. Some people will use a CAM alongside the conventional treatment. Someone else will use the same CAM instead of the approach recommended by their doctor.[4] At the risk of labouring the point, the suggestions below are complementary: they do not replace conventional medicine. And always check with your cancer team before starting a CAM.

Courting controversy

Cancer teams increasingly integrate CAMs into mainstream medi-cine, so-called integrative oncology. Indeed, a growing number of studies suggest that CAMs help some people with cancer. For instance, used alongside conventional treatments, the TCM *Jia Wei Xiao Yao San* prolongs survival in people with liver and breast cancer in clinical studies. The traditional explanation is that it's a 'harmonizing and releasing' formulation.[79, 80] Huang qi (*Astragalus membranaceus*) seems to help breast cancer patients. TCM practi-tioners suggest that huang qi restores the flow of qi around the body.[80] Few conventional Western doctors accept these traditional explanations. They'll look for immune-boosting or cancer-fighting actions on cells.

Cynics, however, point to the lack of evidence supporting many CAMs. Although the evidence is stronger in cancer than for many other diseases, few CAMs undergo the same rigorous testing as modern medicines. But clinical studies are expensive and pharmaceutical companies fund most trials. So, this lack of studies is not surprising. So, no evidence of effectiveness is not necessarily the same as evidence of no effect. In addition, CAMs often combine approaches, which complicates disentangling the benefits of the various treatments.

The placebo response

In other cases, cynics ascribe CAM's benefits to the placebo effect. Indeed, the *placebo response* – the term derives from the Latin phrase 'I shall please' – contributes to the effectiveness of every conventional drug you take, even in cancer, every CAM or psychotherapy you try, every lifestyle change you make.

The placebo response can be remarkably potent. A surgeon operating near the front line during the Korean War began suffering severe abdominal pain, which he knew indicated acute appendicitis. As incoming wounded needed his help, he asked the nurse to give him a morphine injection. The pain eased and he kept working. With the crisis over, the doctor underwent surgery to remove his appendix.[81] After returning to duty, the doctor was looking through the operating room records and found that 'since he appeared distressed' the nurse had injected inactive saline and not morphine.[81] (She probably wanted to avoid the mental fogging that morphine can cause.) In other words, a simple salt solution used to mix injectable drugs alleviated the severe pain of acute appendicitis. Critically, however, the surgeon *expected* the nurse to follow his instructions. He *expected* to receive morphine. This expectation invoked the placebo response – his mind and body reacted as if he had received the morphine. Again, we're beginning to understand how these benefits emerge. For example, placebos can increase levels of the body's natural painkillers and counter anxiety.

In addition, you'll almost certainly get a 'better quality' and longer consultation with a CAM practitioner than with the average pressurized doctor or nurse. The CAM therapist will ask detailed questions about your medical history, diet, lifestyle, sleeping patterns, likes and dislikes, and so on. This offers you the opportunity to talk in detail about yourself and the issues you face to a sympathetic person. Not surprisingly, some people find the consultation therapeutic and their sense of well-being improves.[7] This can bolster the placebo response. Indeed, the quality of your consultation with doctors and nurses also influences the placebo response to conventional medicines.

Spontaneous remissions

Many people with cancer and their carers pray for a miracle. Sometimes their prayers seem to be answered. A cancer may enter remission even when conventional doctors have run out of options. Once again we're beginning to understand how these 'miraculous' spontaneous remissions occur: in many cases, the mind seems to stimulate an immune response that attacks the cancer. (In some ways, it's a supercharged placebo effect.) It's less clear, however, why this immune response only occurs in some people. (If you believe in a higher power, you can think of this as 'how' your prayers were answered.)

Some spontaneous remissions last for years. For example, spontaneous remissions in renal cell carcinoma – a malignancy in the kidney – have lasted between 3 months and 20 years. Nevertheless, most patients relapse[82] and a spontaneous regression is only rarely a cure. On the other hand, metastatic cancer is generally incurable. In many advanced cancers, even the most effective modern treatment usually only buys you time.

Spontaneous remissions are more common than many patients (and probably doctors and nurses) realize and seem to occur in almost every type of cancer.[82] Nevertheless, many doctors seem unwilling to 'recognize, appreciate, and investigate' spontaneous remissions.[83] As a result, 'massive under-reporting' hinders attempts to work out how often spontaneous remissions occur. However, studies suggest that between 1 in every 100,000 and more than 1 in 10,000 cancers might spontaneously enter remission.[83] According to Cancer Research UK, doctors diagnosed 338,623 people with cancer during 2011. So, between 3 and 30 of these may show spontaneous remission. Interestingly, about two-thirds of patients

experienced 'some kind of spiritual awakening' before the spontaneous remission, suggesting that patients had 'a central role in the
process of healing'.[83]

Spontaneous remissions probably account for the case histories
of remarkable cures used by some alternative practitioners. The
combination of CAM and conventional treatment still generally
offers the best long-term prospects. But the intimate link between
mental state and the body underscored by the spontaneous remissions show that while you need to be realistic it's important to
never give up hope.

CAMS for cancer

The rest of this chapter looks at some CAMs that might make your
cancer journey easier. It's not intended to be comprehensive. Given
the large number of CAMs, it's important to take advice from your
cancer team or patient group and to read up on the approach you
want to try. It's worth making the effort: the following examples
illustrate that CAMs can help as part of a holistic approach to
cancer survivorship.

Acupuncture

Acupuncture is one of the best supported CAMs for cancer. And it
may be one of the longest established: archaeologists have uncov-
ered sharpened stones dating from 10,000 BC that they believe were
used for acupuncture. The first texts about acupuncture are probably more than 2,000 years old.

Traditional acupuncture is based on a theory that 12 intercon-
nected channels called meridians connect the body's organs and
internal systems. According to TCM practitioners, qi flows along
these meridians. Stimulating these channels – such as by inserting
a needle – restores the normal balance and flow of qi.[7] Acupressure
stimulates the same points using finger pressure rather than a
needle.[44]

Acupuncture is a well-established treatment for numerous
painful conditions. For instance, a paper in a prestigious medical
journal – the *Archives of Internal Medicine* – considered 31 studies
and reported that acupuncture roughly halved the intensity of
chronic pain caused by back, neck and shoulder problems; osteo-

arthritis; and headache. Yet, the paper points out, 'there is no accepted mechanism by which [acupuncture] could have persisting effects on chronic pain'.[84] Furthermore, scientific studies suggest that, for example:[56, 85]

- acupuncture and acupressure delayed the start and decreased the intensity of nausea and the amount of vomiting in people taking chemotherapy;
- acupuncture and acupressure can alleviate stress and anxiety;
- acupuncture and acupressure may increase energy and physical activity in people receiving chemotherapy;
- acupuncture may help bladder discomfort during radiotherapy;
- acupuncture seems to be promising against fatigue, although more studies are needed.

These are only examples. A qualified acupuncturist will help you decide how they might be able to address your problems.

Art and music therapy

For some people, listening to music is one of the best ways to relax, unwind and deal with illness and other stressors. Some people, for example, find that listening to music before and during chemotherapy helps them cope with the stress of the procedure and reduce discomfort. Indeed, music produces measurable changes in the body – including lowering blood pressure, heart rate and respiration – that indicate reduced stress.[44]

Music therapy takes this a step further and uses singing, playing an instrument, drumming or listening to music to explore and cope with your feelings and emotions about your cancer, treatment and prospects. Music therapy may reduce anxiety and pain, and alleviate some chemotherapy side effects, such as nausea and vomiting.[44]

During art therapy you use paint, clay, collage, sand or writing poetry to help you express and understand your feelings. It works even if you are not artistic: it's for your benefit, it's not going to be displayed in an art gallery. Art therapy can release pent up emotions, relieve stress, bolster your coping skills and help you identify issues that you need to resolve.[44]

Aromatherapy

Your sense of smell may not be anywhere near as sensitive as your dog's or cat's. But it's still powerful: many people find that a distinctive smell can evoke childhood memories, for example. Smell helps make food appetizing or, indeed, can trigger nausea and vomiting.

Aromatherapy uses smells to help improve well-being and quality of life as well as tackling specific problems. For example, some people (not just cancer survivors) find that aromatherapy alleviates depression, stress and tiredness. Lavender, for example, may help alleviate sleeping problems, muscle tension and anxiety. Sweet orange can reduce anxiety.[86] More specifically, aromatherapy can help people take chemotherapy and may reduce the need for other treatments, such as laxatives or painkillers.[4] These are just examples. Aromatherapy books are packed with other conditions and problems that this CAM can alleviate.

The essentials of aromatherapy

Aromatherapy uses oils containing concentrated essences taken from flowers, fruit, seeds, leaves, root or bark. You can use these *essential oils* in various ways, depending on your problem. You can, for example, burn the essential oil or use a diffuser. You can also use essential oils in massage, compresses or baths. You can apply the oil to acupuncture points or as embrocation – a lotion that alleviates muscle or joint pain.[44]

There are more than 400 essential oils, some of which are blends. Essential oils commonly used by people with cancer include frankincense, niaouli, peppermint, lavender, cypress, lemongrass, tea tree oil and marjoram. These are diluted in a carrier, such as grapeseed or apricot oil.[44]

As ever, check first with your cancer team and make sure your aromatherapist knows that you have cancer and your particular problems. Some oils can irritate sensitive skin, for example, or increase sensitivity to sun. Some plant products contain chemicals similar to oestrogen. You shouldn't use these if your malignancy is hormone sensitive. Other oils may interfere with some chemotherapy drugs.[44] It's best to consult a qualified aromatherapist.

Biofeedback

Biofeedback allows you to influence parts of your body that usually work without conscious control, such as heartbeat, blood pressure, respiration rate and muscle tension. Biofeedback machines and software typically make a sound or show a display that varies according to the activity of, for example, your heartbeat. By listening to the sounds or watching the display, practitioners train themselves to regulate the signals. This allows them to exert some control over the body's unconscious functions. Biofeedback helps several problems that can occur in cancer, including urinary incontinence in women, anxiety, pain and constipation.

Counselling and cognitive behavioural therapy

You will have a lot to deal with during your cancer journey – and counselling can help you along the way. Counsellors can help you clarify your problems associated with cancer and more widely, identify the impact on your life and those around you, and devise approaches to tackle issues. So, counselling and CBT can help:

- increase survivors' ability to perform everyday tasks;
- reduce feelings of breathlessness;
- tackle depression, anxiety and stress linked to cancer and more widely;
- counter fatigue and sleep problems;
- enhance general well-being;
- alleviate nausea, constipation, diarrhoea and pain.

In some ways, a therapist is a comforting, supportive friend. However, therapists have no preconceptions or agenda. They make no judgements about you. Unlike talking to family or friends, your choices do not affect the therapist's life. So, their insights, combined with their experience and training, mean that they usually offer more objective and practical help than chatting to a friend.[75] Therapists don't replace your family and friends, of course. Both offer potentially helpful insights and suggestions, but from different perspectives.

Cognitive behavioural therapy

In 1976, the American psychiatrist Aaron Beck suggested that fear and anxiety arise when a person 'senses' danger and they anticipate that they or a loved one could come to harm. Depression arises from a feeling that you have lost something important forever.[87] So, it is hardly surprising that anxiety and depression are common among cancer survivors. You feel happy, in contrast, when you experience enjoyment or expect a pleasurable or positive event.[87] That's one reason why it's important to set goals and plans: you maximize your opportunities for pleasurable, positive experiences.

Beck believed that events do not *directly* cause anxiety, depression and other emotional problems. Rather, our interpretation determines whether we develop anxiety, depression or another psychiatric problem. When you're depressed or anxious, you may interpret a minor symptom as 'proof' that your cancer is progressing or has relapsed. Pain seems worse when you're depressed or anxious. You're less likely to plan to tackle fatigue or take your medicine as suggested by the cancer team. Negative emotions and expectations feed off each other, exacerbating depression or anxiety.[87]

Beck's theory forms the foundation of CBT, which identifies unhelpful feelings, thoughts and behaviours. Your therapist may, for instance, ask you to record negative thoughts and behaviours around cancer or other life events in a diary. You work together to understand how these trigger stress, anxiety, depression, fatigue, poor adherence and so on. You can then look at the evidence for and against each thought and behaviour. Finally, you replace counterproductive ideas with more objective, efficient and effective approaches.[5]

So, CBT and counselling may help you, for instance, prioritize and schedule activities to conserve your energy, improve your coping skills, problem solving and decision making, and enhance your ability to speak to the cancer team, such as offering information rather than waiting to be asked. Therapists may add other elements, such mindfulness and relaxation therapy, which allow you to cope better when faced with a situation that provokes anxiety.

Hypnosis

For centuries, conventional doctors dismissed hypnotism as a stage trick, its benefits confined to weak-willed, gullible people. Some doctors even suggested that subjects 'faked' responses to please their hypnotist.

Yet in the early nineteenth century, there were no effective anaesthetics. Patients usually needed to be drunk and tied down before the surgeon operated. Then, in 1829, the French doctor Pierre-Jean Chapelain used hypnosis as an anaesthetic during a mastectomy for breast cancer. In the 1840s, James Esdaile, a Scottish surgeon working near Calcutta, removed a scrotal tumour using hypnosis as anaesthesia.[88, 89] It is hard to believe someone would endure the pain of a mastectomy or scrotal operation just to please the surgeon. Today, we have powerful painkillers and anaesthetics. (Anaesthetics arrived during the 1840s.) But these examples show hypnotism's power.

Doctors don't fully understand how hypnotism works. Essentially, however, hypnosis is focused attention and concentration.[70, 89] Some hypnotists describe the process as similar to being 'so lost in a book or movie that it is easy to lose track of what is going on around you'.[89] Dissociation (you move competing stimuli to the edge of your awareness) and suggestibility (you go along with the hypnotist's suggestion) probably contribute.

While the mechanism is unclear, many people find that hypnotism helps them to cope with cancer. Hypnotists can suggest, for example, that the cancer survivor will experience less pain, fatigue, distress, nausea and vomiting. Hypnotists can provide coping strategies, such as replacing pain with a numb or cool sensation, or nausea with relaxation.[70, 89] They may construct post-hypnotic suggestions that take effect when you encounter a trigger, such as 'Rubbing your throat with your fingers eliminates any feelings of nausea or discomfort'.[70] Hypnosis can also help change harmful habits such as abusing alcohol, comfort eating or smoking.

Hypnosis is safe. You won't lose control: a hypnotist can't make you do or say anything he or she wants. You'll be able to come 'out' of hypnosis whenever you want.[89] Some people also find that self-hypnosis helps. Numerous DVDs, CDs and books help you create the 'focused attention' that underpins hypnosis.

Guided imagery and visualization

As the occasional spontaneous remissions show, the mind and body are intimately intertwined. Sports people know this: they improve their performance by imagining the goal going in, how they'll win the race or make the try or hit a six.

Essentially, the images 'serve as a bridge between the mind and body'. Guided imagery and visualization use your imagination to change your body, mind and emotions and help you cope with cancer.[44] So, you might visualize immune cells attacking cancer cells or a soothing feeling around a sore part of your body. You might visualize a 'safe place' (it can be a made-up place or a favourite haunt) when you're undergoing an uncomfortable procedure or receiving chemotherapy. This helps cut stress and anxiety. The more you call the image to mind, the stronger the image and the greater the benefit will be.

Guided imagery takes visualization a step further. During guided imagery you use imagery, metaphor, story-telling, fantasy exploration and game playing. You can do this on your own – several books can teach you the principles – although many people find having a therapist guide the internal journey helps.

In people with cancer, guided imagery and visualization may improve energy, sleep and digestion, and counter stress, anxiety, pain and fatigue. Guided imagery and visualization might boost the immune system, ease symptoms and side effects, speed recovery from surgery and improve emotional control.[44]

Tai chi and qi gong

Tai chi (*tai chi chuan*) is a 'soft' or 'internal' martial art that combines deep breathing, meditation and relaxation with sequences (called forms) of slow gentle movements that enhance fitness, strength and flexibility. As such tai chi is often suitable (after checking with your doctor) for people with cancer and other long-term diseases.

Tai chi's slow, gentle movements improve strength, balance, posture, concentration, relaxation and breath control. So, tai chi helps prevent falls and improves how well your heart and lungs work.[90] Researchers examined 33 studies evaluating tai chi in people with cancer, osteoarthritis, heart failure or chronic obstructive pulmonary disease. Across these diseases, tai chi improved physical performance.[90]

Tai chi may look undemanding until you try it. You can learn the tai chi short form in about 12 lessons. However, tai chi takes many years to master. Speeded up, tai chi can offer effective self-defence – indeed, *chuan* means 'fist'. Speed up a raising hand and you may deflect a blow to the head, while a descending hand can deflect a kick.

Qi gong also combines deep breathing, meditation, relaxation and movements. However, the movements are more internally focused on the 'flow of energy' around the body than tai chi.

Herbal medicines

Plants provide invaluable sources of painkillers and 'conventional' cancer drugs: morphine, a mainstay of cancer pain management, comes from a poppy and has been used for thousands of years.

In 1962, a botanist named Arthur Barclay peeled some bark from a Pacific Yew tree (*Taxus brevifolia*) growing in the Gifford Pinchot National Forest in north-eastern USA.[91] Today, oncologists use a drug called paclitaxel, extracted from the yew's bark, to treat various malignancies including lung, breast and ovarian cancer.[91] The small, pink-violet Madagascar periwinkle (*Catharanthus roseus*) yielded a drug called vincristine, which has helped improve the chances of surviving childhood leukaemia from less than 10 per cent in 1960 to more than 90 per cent today. Indeed, almost half of cancer drugs introduced between the 1940s and 2010 are natural products or their direct derivatives.[92]

Conventional drugs from natural sources tend to use a single chemical isolated from the plant. Originally, chemists needed the bark from 100 trees to yield just one gram of paclitaxel, for example.[12] Herbalists use the whole plant or part of a plant – the root, leaf and so on. Herbalists believe that various chemicals in a plant act together to increase effectiveness – so-called synergy. Some components work together to reduce the risk of side effects – buffering. Using several plants together, according to herbalists, further increases activity and buffering.[7] This idea is similar to that underlying combinations of chemotherapy drugs.

This makes identifying which chemicals are responsible for the benefits difficult, especially if they act synergistically. For example, the traditional herbal Chinese herbal remedies *Jia Wei Xiao Yao San* and *Chai Hu Shu Gan Tang* prolong survival in people with liver cancer when used alongside conventional treatments. They contain ten and seven plants respectively.[79] And each plant potentially produces hundreds of biologically active chemicals.

Herbal help for people with cancer

Many herbs could potentially help people with cancer. For example, in people with breast cancer, mistletoe may improve survival, enhance quality of life and reduce the risk of side effects of chemotherapy, when used alongside conventional treatments. Indeed, numerous studies suggest that extracts of mistletoe have anti-cancer actions.[93] However, mistletoe is poisonous and you should use this only under medical supervision.

Milk thistle (*Silybum marianum*), a member of the same botanical family as daisies and sunflowers, grows wild across southern Europe, southern Russia, Asia Minor and North Africa. Since antiquity, European healers have used milk thistle to treat liver and gall bladder disorders. The extract of milk thistle used commonly, called silymarin, contains four chemicals. One of these – silibinin (silybin) – accounts for about 50 to 70 per cent of silymarin. Experimental studies suggest that silibinin alone and silymarin, among other actions, mop up tissue-damaging free radicals, counter inflammation and may directly kill cancer cells, which boosts the effectiveness of conventional chemotherapies.[94]

The Ancient Egyptians, Greeks and Romans used chamomile to alleviate conditions as diverse as colds, sore throats, abscesses, eczema, anxiety and insomnia. Camomile tea contains a chemical called apigenin, which is a mild sedative. Herbalists may suggest chamomile as an anti-inflammatory, or to boost immunity, alleviate anxiety, treat diarrhoea or facilitate sleep.[95] Valerian is another 'classic' herbal remedy to improve fatigue, reduce drowsiness and alleviate problems sleeping.[5] But like any drug, it's best to use these for only a few weeks while sleep hygiene (page 72) begins to restore a restful night.

A traditional Chinese medicine – a soup called *Ren Shen Yangrong Tang* – may help with cancer-related fatigue. *Ren Shen Yangrong Tang* contains 12 herbs including ginseng or dang shen (*Codonopsis pilosula*, sometimes called the poor man's ginseng) and huang qi. In one study of survivors who had completed their conventional cancer treatment, *Ren Shen Yangrong Tang* roughly halved fatigue severity. Twenty-two patients reported severe fatigue before TCM. After drinking *Ren Shen Yangrong Tang* twice a day for six weeks, 11 had mild fatigue and 11 had moderate fatigue.[96]

On the other hand, certain herbs cause side effects and some interact with conventional drugs that you are taking for cancer or another problem. So, always check with your cancer team before taking a herbal remedy. Ideally, see a qualified medical herbalist or TCM practitioner and let them know which conventional treatment you are taking rather than buy supplements from a health food shop. Be very careful buying herbs (or conventional medicines) over the net unless you are absolutely sure of the source.

Traditional Chinese medicines and cancer

Numerous studies suggest that TCM can help tackle certain cancers, such as the following.

- Used alongside conventional treatments by patients with liver cancer, TCM improved survival by more than a third (35 per cent).[79]
- TCM, again combined with conventional treatments, improved survival in women with advanced breast cancer by about half: 45 per cent for those taking TCM between for 30 and 180 days and by 54 per cent if used for more than 180 days.[80]
- In head and neck cancer, TCM plus conventional treatments improved survival by a third (32 per cent). Using TCM for between 251 and 550 days (about 18 months) improved survival by two-fifths (43 per cent) and by almost three-quarters (70 per cent) for those taking TCM for more than 550 days.[97]

Active relaxation and progressive muscular relaxation

As a way to relax, there is nothing wrong with curling up with a good book or watching your favourite television programme or DVD. However, many of us, not just people with cancer, need to take a more 'active' approach to relaxation. The following tips should help. You may need to adapt these if, for example, you want to meditate or practise yoga.

- Find time for your relaxation therapy every day. Many people find that the early morning is best for 'active relaxation'. The house is quiet and you will be better able to focus and less likely to drop off to sleep than later at night.

- Sit in a comfortable chair that supports your back or lie down. You might want to put cushions under your neck and knees. Take off your shoes, switch off bright lights and ensure the room is a comfortable temperature.
- Do not try to perform relaxation therapy on a full stomach. After a meal, blood diverts from your muscles to your stomach. Trying progressive muscle relaxation (see below) on a full stomach can cause cramps. And relaxation can make you more aware of your body's functions. A full stomach can be a distraction.
- Shut your eyes and, if it helps, play some relaxing music and burn some aromatherapy oils.

Then follow your relaxation regimen, such as guided imagery or meditation. Alternatively, try progressive muscular relaxation (PMR).

- Put your hands by your side. You can stand, sit or lie down. Now clench your fists as hard as you can. Hold the fist for ten seconds.
- Now slowly relax your fist and let your hands hang or rest on the floor loosely by your sides. Then shrug your shoulders as high as you can. Hold for ten seconds and then relax slowly.
- Now gently arch your back, hold for ten seconds and relax. Tense your muscles as you inhale. Don't hold your breath. Try to breathe slowly and rhythmically.
- Exhale as you relax.
- Repeat each exercise three times, slowly, gently and gradually.

Most PMR teachers advise mastering one muscle group at a time. It could take two or three months before you can tense and relax your entire body. Speak to your doctor before trying PMR if you have muscle, joint or skeletal problems, because of your cancer, your treatment or another ailment.

Massage

Many people with cancer find that massage alleviates pain, anxiety, nausea and fatigue while improving general well-being. In one study, for example, massage seemed to alleviate anxiety (60 per cent improvement), nausea (51 per cent), depression (49 per cent), pain (48 per cent) and fatigue (43 per cent). People who are too weak for normal Swedish massage (57 per cent improvement in symptoms overall) might still benefit from light-touch massage (62 per cent) or foot (50 per cent) massage.[98] Many cancer patients report that hot stone massage is particularly beneficial.[44]

Moreover, in patients with acute myelogenous leukaemia gentle massage reduced stress, improved quality of life, relaxation and comfort and made hospital stays 'more tolerable'.[99] The improvement in blood circulation produced by massage can, some CAM practitioners suggest, aid cellular replacement, promote digestion and act as a detoxifier. Whether or not this is the case, massage certainly reduces depression, stress and anxiety, improves muscle tone, mobility and pain, as well as fostering a sense of relaxation and well-being.[44]

Make sure you consult an experienced masseur and check with the cancer team first. Inappropriate pressure, for example, can cause pain and joint or tissue manipulation may not be suitable for some survivors. Some healthcare professionals think that massage near a tumour could promote the cancer's spread. Until studies clarify any risk, it's probably prudent to avoid massage close to a malignancy. It also best to avoid massage if your skin is broken, you have open wounds, a rash, blood clots, broken bones or osteoporosis.[44]

Meditation, prayer and mindfulness

Essentially, mindfulness and meditation encourage you to concentrate, non-judgementally and openly, on the present rather than worry about what might happen or ruminate on the past. Mindfulness and meditation allow you a step back from your anxiety, depression, stress and other emotions associated with cancer and more generally. As such, mindfulness and meditation seem to increase your ability to regulate your behaviour, thoughts and emotions, as well as improving the flexibility of your thinking and enhancing attention. Mindfulness and meditation are a bit like waking up from life spent on automatic pilot.

In people with cancer, for example, a mindfulness-based stress-reduction programme can help reduce fears about recurrence, anxiety and depression, improve energy levels and enhance the survivor's ability to perform everyday tasks.[5] One study compared mindfulness-based stress reduction over 8 weeks with education and support in survivors of breast or colorectal cancer experiencing moderate or severe fatigue. Both approaches improved cognitive performance after 8 weeks and 6 months. The improvement was, however, greater with mindfulness.[100]

Learning classical meditation or mindfulness can be difficult without face-to-face guidance; you could see if your local adult education centres or other local groups hold courses. But to get a taste of mindfulness or mediation, focus on a single object, idea, subject or sensation. If you mind wanders off, bring it back to your focus. Try not to get annoyed if you fail. This is often much more difficult than it sounds. Mindfulness encourages you to become more aware of your body and its response to internal and external stimuli.[101] However, people with cancer may already be highly sensitive to mental and physical changes. So, try not to become preoccupied with how you feel.

In many ways, mindfulness is similar to the early stages of the mediation techniques taught by Buddhism and some other Eastern religions and certain types of prayer, but stripped of religious connotations. Indeed, meditation is not confined to sitting in the lotus position for hours chanting 'om' or another mantra: most people find it easier to be more aware while walking or moving. Tai chi, qi gong, yoga and rosary prayer are forms of meditation. Your vicar or spiritual adviser can offer advice about prayer.

Yoga

Yoga brings millions of people – from all religious backgrounds – inner peace, relief from stress and improved health. Yoga aims to harmonize consciousness, mind, energy and body. (The Indian root of the word 'yoga' means 'to unite'.)

Essentially, yoga focuses on achieving controlled, slow, deep breaths, while the poses (*asanas*) increase fitness, strength and flexibility. As a result, yoga helps maintain suppleness of both body and mind (some poses require considerable concentration).

Clinical studies suggest that yoga may alleviate anxiety, headaches, depression, back and neck pain, and several other conditions. Indeed, yoga improves mood and reduces anxiety more than the same time spent walking.[102] In another study, people who took part in three hour-long yoga sessions a week for 12 weeks showed greater improvements in anxiety, tranquillity and 'revitalization' than those who burnt the same calories off walking.[103]

In cancer survivors, yoga seems to reduce anxiety, distress and fatigue, while improving quality of life, and emotional and social functioning, and protecting against cancer-related cognitive impairment.[36] Researchers looked at 16 studies of breast cancer survivors. People who took part in yoga showed improved overall quality of life, depression, anxiety and gastrointestinal symptoms. Some benefits might take time to emerge, however. For example, improvements in anxiety only emerged after practising yoga for longer than three months.[104] Always let your yoga tutor know that you currently have or have survived cancer and any particular problems. This helps them make sure the *asanas* are right for you.

Think about your breathing

One of the first things that a yoga, martial arts or meditation teacher will probably tell you is that you are not breathing correctly. Most of us breathe shallowly, using the upper parts of our lungs. Try putting one hand on your chest and the other on your abdomen. Then breathe normally. Most people find that the hand on their chest moves while the one on the abdomen remains relatively still. To fill your lungs completely, try to make the hand on your abdomen rise, while keeping the one on the chest as still as possible.

Breathing deeply and slowly without gasping helps you relax. If you feel stressed out try breathing in deeply through your nose for the count of four, hold your breath for a count of seven; then breathe out for a count of eight. Repeat a dozen times.

Using CAMs safely

If you want to try a CAM, check with your cancer team first and consult a registered practitioner, such as one recognized by the General Regulatory Council for Complementary Therapies or the Complementary and Natural Healthcare Council. Read up on the approach you are planning to use – this chapter is a general introduction – and make sure you understand the risks and benefits. Make sure that the CAM practitioner knows you have cancer and your current and previous treatments. Ideally, the CAM practitioner should be experienced in treating people with cancer. You could ask your cancer team if they know of a practitioner.

Watch for side effects. For example, some alternative healers believe that CAMs drive out toxins that have accumulated in your body. They say that this toxic 'tsunami' can produce a detox 'crisis', characterized by, for example, headaches, fatigue and abdominal discomfort. In some cases, the healer and the person undergoing detox can dismiss adverse events as a symptom of the detox crisis. So, you need to be careful if you experience any unexpected symptoms.

Keep an eye on whether or not the CAM is working. You could keep a diary to track the improvement over 3–4 months and then speak to the CAM and cancer team if you feel it's not working. It's important not to feel that you've failed. And, if you're sticking to their suggestions, don't be tempted to adhere even more robustly to the CAM. There is probably a better approach for you at this stage in your cancer journey.

As stressed before, never believe claims that a particular CAM can cure a cancer or follow advice to stop a conventional therapy or eat a highly restricted diet. Often the CAM practitioner is acting with the best of intentions. However, your best chance comes from using CAMs as part of a holistic approach alongside conventional treatments, a healthy balanced diet and an anti-cancer lifestyle, which we'll discuss in the next chapter.

6

An anti-cancer lifestyle

According to Cancer Research UK, a healthy lifestyle would have prevented two in every five (42 per cent) malignaucies. But it's never too late to improve your chances: a healthy lifestyle may protect against recurrence or second primary malignancies.

Despite cancer never being far from the headlines, many people seem unaware of the link between lifestyle and malignancies. A 2015 survey for the World Cancer Research Fund found that about two-fifths of adults in Britain are unaware of the increased cancer risk linked to poor diets (40 per cent unaware), being overweight (41 per cent) or alcohol (43 per cent). More than half (54 per cent) are not aware that physical inactivity can increase cancer risk.

This chapter considers quitting smoking, exercise and controlling alcohol consumption as part of an anti-cancer lifestyle. We'll also take a look at the social supports that can help you along your cancer journey.

Quit smoking

According to Action on Smoking and Health (ASH), smoking in Great Britain peaked in 1948 when 82 per cent of men smoked. By 1974, 45 per cent of adults smoked. By 2015, according to the Smoking Toolkit Study, 19 per cent of adults smoked.

There is, typically, a 20-year delay between smoking and the emergence of lung cancer. So, the number of smoking-related cancers is lagging someway behind these encouraging reductions. Smoking caused 86 per cent of lung cancers in the UK in 2010 as well as, among other malignancies: 65 per cent of cancers in the mouth, throat and oesophagus; 29 per cent of pancreatic cancers; and 22 per cent of stomach cancers.[105] Overall, smokers are roughly twice as likely to die from cancer as non-smokers.

On the other hand, quitting reduces your likelihood of developing most smoking-related diseases. It's even worth quitting if you already have cancer. A study of people with advanced lung cancer found that continuing to smoke undermined quality of life, for example.[106] Another study found that people who quit smoking after being diagnosed with lung cancer were about seven times more likely to maintain a better performance status during the year-long study than those who continued to smoke, even allowing for factors such as treatment and disease stage.[107]

The dangers to your family

Second-hand smoke contains more than 4000 chemicals, including about 50 carcinogens. This chemical cocktail increases the risk that people who inhale second-hand smoke will develop serious diseases, including cancer, heart disease, asthma and sudden infant death syndrome. Over a lifetime, passive smokers inhale a similar amount of fine particle 'pollution' as non-smokers living in heavily polluted cities, such as Beijing.[108]

Making quitting easier

On some measures, nicotine is more addictive than heroin or cocaine. As a result, fewer than 1 in 30 smokers quit annually and many relapse within a year, partly because of withdrawal symptoms, which include feeling irritable, restless and anxious; insomnia; and enduring intense cravings for a cigarette.

Typically, withdrawal symptoms abate over two weeks or so. If you cannot tough it out, nicotine replacement therapy (NRT) 'tops up' levels and reduces withdrawal symptoms, without exposing you to other harmful chemicals. NRT increases your chance of quitting by between 50 per cent and 100 per cent. But you need to find the right combination for you. Patches alleviate withdrawal symptoms for 16 to 24 hours, but begin to work relatively slowly. Nicotine chewing gum, lozenges, inhalers and nasal spray act more quickly, but don't last as long. Talk to your pharmacist, nurse or GP to find out which is right for you. Doctors can prescribe other treatments, such as bupropion and varenicline, that help you quit.

Electronic cigarettes (also called vaping) also help many people quit. The nicotine staves off withdrawal symptoms and means you are not exposed to the chemicals that cause cancer and other dis-eases linked to tobacco. In part, ASH suggests, vaping's success may reflect e-cigarettes' ability to replicate smoking's superficial aspects. Even placebo e-cigarettes, which don't contain nicotine, reduce cravings, alleviate withdrawal and cut cigarette consumption. The wide range of e-cigarettes means that you should be able to find one that suits you.

However, e-cigarettes can cause mouth and throat irritation, and any long-term side effects are poorly characterized. So, it's best to use e-cigarettes to stop rather than replace smoking. In addition, the risks from passive vaping to non-smokers are not fully understood, so it might be prudent to limit passive exposure as far as practical.

Tips to help you quit

NRT and e-cigarettes help you quit. But you need to be motivated and tackle any issues that maintain your habit. For example, smoking seems to offer some smokers a 'sense of control' and a way to 'fill a void created by a lack of meaningful activities'.[109] So, keep a diary of problems and situations that tempt you to light up – such as stress, boredom, a low mood, anxiety and worries, coffee, meals and pubs. Then find an alternative. If you find yourself smoking when you get home in the evening, try a new hobby. If it's pressure at work, anxiety or depression, try stress-management, mindfulness or active relaxation. If you find car journeys boring without a cigarette, try an audio book. A few other hints may make life easier.

- Hypnosis can increase the chances of quitting smoking almost five-fold.[89]
- Not letting other people smoke in your home helps strengthen your resolve.
- Try to quit abruptly. People who cut back the number of cigarettes they smoke usually inhale more deeply to get the same amount of nicotine. Reduction takes you a step towards kicking the habit – but don't stop there.
- Set a quit date. Smokers are more likely to quit if they set a specific date rather than saying, for example, that they will give up in the next two months.
- Smoking is expensive. Keep a note of how much you save and spend at least some of it on something for yourself.
- Get a free 'quit smoking' pack from the NHS online (at: www.nhs.uk/smokefree/help-and-advice/support) or the Smokefree National Helpline (0300 123 1044).

- Your local stop smoking service offers support and advice about NRT and other aspects of quitting. People who use the service with NRT are up to four times more likely to quit than those who just try to stop. Speaking to an adviser before your quit date can help you cope with withdrawal symptoms.
- Watch your drinking. Abstinence from drinking seems to improve your chances of quitting and heavy drinkers are more likely than light or moderate drinkers to continue smoking after a diagnosis of cancer.[110] Alcohol can, after all, sap willpower.

Dealing with setbacks

Nicotine is incredibly addictive. So, most smokers make three or four attempts to quit before they succeed.[76] Regard any relapse as a temporary setback and try to identify why you relapsed. Were you stressed out, anxious or depressed? Did a particular time, place or event cause you to light up? Once you know why you slipped you can develop strategies to stop the problem. Then set another quit date and try again. As the old health promotion advertisement suggests, 'Don't give up on giving up.'

Drinking

Excessive alcohol consumption increases the risk of developing several malignancies including cancers in the mouth, throat, voice box (larynx), oesophagus, liver, colon and rectum, pancreas and breast. The risk rises with the amount of alcohol you drink. However, even relatively low levels of alcohol can increase the risk: consuming 2.5 units or less a day (20 g) accounts for between a quarter (26 per cent) and a third (35 per cent) of deaths from cancer caused by alcohol.[111] That's less than about a pint of beer, lager or cider or a 250 ml glass of red or white wine.

The increased risk of cancer linked to alcohol seems to be especially high among smokers. Heavy drinking, smoking or both seems to account for about three-quarters of upper aerodigestive tract cancers (malignancies of the lips, mouth, tongue, nose, throat, vocal cords, and parts of the oesophagus and trachea).[110] The combination seems to be especially hazardous. Alcohol seems to dissolve some carcinogens in smoke, increasing the amount that reaches and damages the tissue.

Nevertheless, studies assessing whether continuing to drink increases the risk of recurrence after you have survived a cancer reported mixed results. There's theoretical grounds for concern: alcohol may raise levels of some hormones, for example. Moreover, drinking may increase the risk that you will develop an alcohol-related second primary cancer or be at increased risk of complications following surgery or radiotherapy. For instance, a study of people with upper aerodigestive tract cancers found that:

- continuing to drink after diagnosis increases the risk of complications during and after surgery between two and four times;
- the risk of death due to complications, such as sepsis and pneumonia, was three times higher in people who abuse alcohol after surgery to remove the tumour;
- the risk of second primary malignancies was 50 per cent higher in those with upper aerodigestive tract cancers who consumed more than 24 units a week, after allowing for smoking.

Other studies suggest that the increased risk of second primary malignancies may be at least three times higher (i.e., 300 per cent) for certain upper aerodigestive tract cancers in those who continued to drink.[110]

Alcohol, even in small amounts, may irritate and exacerbate mouth sores caused by some cancer treatments. In addition, alcohol can interact with some cancer treatments, which can increase the risk of side effects. So, check with your cancer team whether and how much you can drink during treatment and the limits following your diagnosis. Always follow the cancer team's advice: your limit may differ from the government's recommendation.

You might also find that you use alcohol to help you cope as you live with cancer or deal with the aftermath. If you are worried you're going over your cancer team's recommendation or feel you're drinking too much, keep a note of how much you drink and don't just guess. According to Alcohol Concern, the average adult drinker underestimates their consumption by a bottle of wine each week (a 750 ml bottle of 12 per cent wine contains nine units). You may find that keeping track means that you start cutting down. If you get so drunk that you cannot recall how much you drank the night before, you need to cut back.

If you find that you drink to alleviate the stress of cancer, speak to your cancer team or GP, who can refer you to NHS Alcohol Services, or to a counsellor. Psychotherapy can help you understand why you drink, how to cut down and how to deal with difficult situations.

Simple tips to help you cut back

- Replace large glasses with smaller ones.
- Use a measure at home rather than guess how many units you're pouring.
- Avoid wine with alcohol by volume (ABV) of 14 per cent or 15 per cent. Buy 10 per cent ABV or less.
- Alternate alcoholic and soft drinks.
- Try spritzers and shandies rather than wine and beer.
- Quench your thirst with a soft drink rather than an alcoholic beverage.
- Have several drink-free days each week. You may need to avoid your usual haunts and drinking partners on dry days.
- Find a hobby that does not involve drinking.
- Groups buying rounds tend to keep pace with the fastest drinker. Buy your own or buy rounds only in small groups.
- If you rely on a nightcap to get to sleep, try the tips on page 72.
- If you drink to drown your sorrows, stress, depression or anxiety, try counselling, mindfulness, active relaxation or hypnosis.

Take regular exercise

You may not always feel up to a workout, especially if you're fatigued, your muscles or joints ache, or you feel depressed. Yet overwhelming evidence shows that regular exercise brings important benefits for cancer survivors,[25, 36, 38, 40, 112] including the following.

- Physical activity is, ironically, one of the best ways to counter fatigue. That's one reason why regular exercise helps you look after yourself and improves quality of life.
- Many people find that exercise alleviates anxiety, depression and stress.
- Exercise may reduce the impact on your body composition from the cancer and its treatment. Exercise, for example, builds stronger muscles and bones, and improves heart and lung function.

- Exercise can help counter nausea and vomiting, sharpen your appetite, improve digestion and prevent constipation.
- Exercise may help prevent and treat lymphoedema, 'menopausal' symptoms linked to hormonal treatments, and cancer-related cognitive impairment.
- Exercise may improve survival. For instance, women with breast cancer who reduced their physical activity after their malignancy was diagnosed were twice as likely to die over the next 11 years than those who maintained or increased exercise.[113]

Speak to your cancer team before beginning exercise or physical activity. You might need to adapt your diet, for example, or you might be vulnerable to certain injuries. For example, people with skeletal metastasis or bone loss due to therapy should avoid activities, such as jumping or twisting the hips, that could increase the risk of fractures. Chemotherapy-induced neuropathy (nerve damage) may affect balance, which means you should exercise in a way that avoids the risk of falls.[38] And make sure you drink enough during exercise to avoid dehydration.

Finding the time to exercise

Unless your cancer team tells you otherwise, try to get at least 30 minutes of moderate physical activity on most, if not all, days. There are many ways to incorporate physical activity into your daily life. For instance, find an exercise that you enjoy and that fits into your lifestyle. If you do not like exercise classes and you join a gym some distance from home or work, you are more likely to quit. On the other hand, you can easily integrate walking or, in some parts of the country, riding a bike into your daily life.

Find a time of day to exercise that suits you. Some people find that exercising in the morning helps them focus better on the day.[114] That's fine if you can jog or cycle to work and can have a shower when you arrive or you can get to an early gym class. However, some people cannot get up early enough (their body clock is more attuned to the evenings that the mornings), have a long commute, the roads are dangerous, or they need to get the kids to school. They would probably be better off exercising in the evening.

There are plenty of other opportunities make exercise part of your day-to-day life, such as the following.

- Clean the house regularly and wash your car by hand.
- Grow your own vegetables – and they taste better.
- If you take the bus, tube, train or metro, get off one or two stops early.
- Park a 15-minute walk from your place of work.
- Use the stairs instead of the lift.
- Walk to the local shops instead of taking the car.
- If you're confined to bed, a physiotherapist could suggest exercises that maintain strength and the joint's range of motion. Prolonged bedrest can reduce fitness, endurance and muscle strength, which can make performing daily activities even more difficult. Even in bed, physical activity can help counteract the fatigue and give you a mental and emotional boost.[38]
- Protect time to exercise in your diary and make exercise part of your daily plan to counter fatigue (page 69).

Get out in nature

The benefits of exercising in nature go beyond the physical alone. Getting out and about in nature – even urban green spaces – reduces stress and anger, improves mental abilities, and enhances happiness and self-esteem. Exercising in nature may even speed recovery from operations and other treatments.

In a now famous study, Roger Ulrich, from Delaware University in the USA, compared the recovery of two groups of patients who had undergone a common type of gall bladder surgery. One group could look out of a window at a small stand of deciduous trees. The other group could see only a brown brick wall. The rooms were otherwise nearly identical and Ulrich allowed for age and other factors that might influence recovery. For example, the same nurses looked after both groups. For several years, Ulrich collected data about patients' recovery between May and October, when the trees had foliage.[115]

People who could see the trees spent, on average, just under a day less in hospital than those who looked at a brick wall. Nurses were about four times less likely to make negative comments in the medical notes – such as 'upset and crying' or 'needs much encouragement' – and more likely to make positive observations – including 'in good spirits' and 'moving well' – about people who looked out on the trees.[115]

Patients with a view of the trees were slightly less likely to experience minor complications – such as nausea and headache – following their operation. The group facing the wall needed many more doses of potent painkillers (such as opioids) than those with a view of trees. In general, those able to look at the trees used less potent analgesics, such as aspirin and paracetamol.[115] So, the view of the trees boosted recovery, and reduced pain and stress.

Japanese people believe that walking in forests promotes physical and mental health. The Japanese term *Shinrin-yoku* – 'forest bathing' – means 'making contact with and taking in the atmosphere of the forest'.[116] Just looking at a picture of people walking in a forest reduces blood pressure, researchers found. However, the smell and other sensations of walking through a forest augment the visual appreciation.[117] As the East Anglian writer Ronald Blythe notes in *From The Headlands* when nature is 'right under our noses, we inhale it as well as comprehending it with our intellects'. You absorb the 'earthy patterns and colours . . . instinctively as well as intellectually'.

Against this background, forest bathers produced less cortisol – a hormone released during stress – and showed lower blood pressure and pulse rates than those who took a similar amount of exercise in towns and cities. Forest bathing also seems to boost immunity. Just walking in a forest for 15 minutes and then sitting for another 15 minutes enhanced feelings of vigour, while reducing depression, tension and anxiety compared to walking and sitting in an urban environment. The benefits were especially marked in people who felt chronic mental stress,[117] which is a problem for many cancer survivors and their carers.

Make the most of your local country parks and nature reserves. If you are worried about tripping, call the reserve in advance or look for those with prepared paths (such as many National Trust properties). The following are good places to start:

- The National Trust <www.nationaltrust.org.uk>
- The Ramblers <www.ramblers.org.uk/go-walking.aspx>
- The Royal Society for the Protection of Birds <www.rspb.org.uk/discoverandenjoynature/seenature/reserves>
- The Woodland Trust <visitwoods.org.uk>.

Ecotherapy

In one study, women with breast cancer cultivated and customized a garden bowl for three months. The women reported that the 'ecotherapy' reflected their cancer journey; inspired positivity; allowed them to discover meaning through memories; and augmented their sense of control.[118] You could try to make bowls and pots of flowers and plants: there is a massive choice of indoor and outdoor plants. You could also use gardening or volunteering at a nature reserve as ecotherapy – and they'll help keep you active.

Spirituality and religion

More than 40,000 years ago, Neanderthal and Palaeolithic man engaged in complex religious rituals, seemed to 'understand' the idea of death and drew images of mythical creatures on cave walls.[119] As John Polkinghorne points out: 'at almost all times and in almost all places, human beings have participated in an admittedly bafflingly diverse history of encounters with the sacred'.[120]

Today, religion and spirituality help many cancer patients find meaning in their illness, provide comfort and engender a sense of purpose. Religious and spiritual groups also offer practical support, including transport, childcare and meals. As cancer is so common, many people in the group have probably dealt with a malignancy as a patient, carer or both. Every cancer, every person, is different. But they may still have insights, suggestions and experiences that can help.

In addition, people who follow and participate in a religion are often healthier than their more secular counterparts. Religious people are, for example, more likely to avoid some lifestyles that increase the risk of certain cancers, such as alcohol abuse, smoking tobacco and having a greater number of sexual partners,[121] which increases the chance of contracting HPV and some other carcinogenic viruses.

Religion and spirituality can foster hope, forgiveness, comfort, love and other emotional benefits and buffer against stress.[121] Moreover, some religions engender a 'respect' for authority, which increases the chances that people will follow their doctor's advice. That might be part of the reason why people who report higher levels of spiritual well-being are more likely to take their medicines as their doctors suggest.[122]

Side effects of religion and spirituality

However, it's not all good news. Some religious people hold unrealistically high expectations for themselves and others. Others may be reluctant to engage with people who do not share their beliefs. This can leave them isolated when they need support. Some people may feel – or be told – that their cancer is God's punishment. Feeling that God is punishing or has abandoned you can increase depression and decrease adherence to medical advice.

You can even have too much faith. Some people seem to 'over-rely' on their relationship with God to aid recovery. This can develop into a form of fatalism,[123] which means people are less likely to follow screening and treatment recommendations. Living a fulfilled life depends on taking an active approach: God helps those who help themselves.

Finally, some religions may advise against medical suggestions, such as immunization, transfusions and treatment with blood products. The final choice is up to you. But speaking to your cancer team and your spiritual leader allows you to make a fully informed decision.

Social networks

Religion, close family and friends can create a sense of community and belonging, which can bolster your mental and physical resources and offer social, practical and emotional support. Indeed, people with strong social connections show less marked changes in blood pressure when they face high levels of negative emotions than those with fewer or weaker networks.[124]

Social networks support your cancer journey in many ways. Your partner's and family's practical and emotional support can be invaluable if you are trying to drink less alcohol, quit smoking, take more exercise, change your diet or take medicines as prescribed. Your partner can help you adopt a healthy lifestyle, ignore bad moods triggered by the disease or lifestyle change, boost your motivation, can watch out for problems – including fatigue, anxiety and depression – and encourage the survivor to see a doctor when they feel unwell, seem to be taking a turn for the worse or could be developing side effects.

So, try to develop relationships that preserve or enhance your emotional well-being and bolster your ability to cope, and disengage from those that are counterproductive. After all, social networks that cause profound stress are hardly good for your mental or physical health. In some cases, such as your family, you may not be able to remove yourself from the network. However, you can probably find ways to limit their influence.

Meanwhile, partners and family members need to tread the fine line between 'nagging' (even with the best intentions) and 'support'. Support helps and reinforces their loved one's efforts to tackle unhealthy behaviours. Control – trying to persuade a partner to adopt healthy behaviours when he or she is unwilling or unable – can reduce the likelihood that the person would make the changes.

A menagerie of therapeutic animals

For centuries, healers have used a menagerie – including dogs, cats, guinea pigs, rabbits and horses – to bolster well-being. Handicapped people in Belgium helped care for farm animals in the ninth century. In the 1700s, the York Retreat used rabbits, seagulls, hawks and other domestic animals to promote well-being in people with mental illness. Florence Nightingale suggested that a small pet 'is often an excellent companion' for ill people, especially those with chronic diseases.[125]

Caring for an animal can, for example, help create a purpose in life and evoke pleasant memories, which help take your mind off your cancer and encourage exercise. Caring for and interacting with animals alleviates stress, which is obviously a major problem for many cancer survivors and their carers. Even a fish tank in a dentist's waiting room reduces anxiety in what many people find an intensely stressful situation.[125] Some people speak more openly to their pet than their spouse, probably because animals are non-judgemental, which helps get problems off the owner's chest. As one of George Eliot's characters remarks: 'Animals are such agreeable friends – they ask no questions, pass no criticisms'.

Towards the end

Telling people that you have cancer or that the malignancy has recurred can be difficult. In turn, family and friends may find discussing cancer difficult. The following suggestions might make these difficult conversations a little easier.

- Minimize distractions – turn the television, radio and phones off.
- Sit comfortably and make sure you can see each person you are speaking to.
- You might find it easier to tell some people (such as acquaintances, rather than close family and friends, and human resources) over the telephone, or by letter or email. You might want to ask someone you have told if they can let others know and tell them what they can share.
- Think about the points you want to make beforehand and make sure you cover everything. Don't be afraid to write a list and refer to it during the discussions.
- Introduce the subject gradually and gently. Ask what they already know. This means you do not need to repeat information. You could also suggest websites and books where they can find out more.
- Give information in small chunks and allow the listeners time for it to sink in. Check that everyone understands: it's easy to miss something important at an emotional time or when you're communicating technical information.
- Do not worry about silences. You, or your relatives or friends, might not know what to say. Hold hands, hug and ask what they are thinking about.
- Do not hide your fears or your feelings and let people know the full situation, including the uncertainties about treatment and prospects. They need the whole picture to help and might feel hurt or confused if they find out later.
- Tell people how much you love them and how grateful you are for their support.
- Telling children and grandchildren can be especially difficult. You will need to tailor the information to their level of understanding and emotional development.

The end arrives quickly for most people with cancer. A person dying from cancer may become bed-bound or semi-comatose. They may be unable to eat normally or take drugs by mouth and only sip water. Confusion, especially at the end of life, is relatively common. The person may, for example, seem disorientated, behave or communicate inappropriately, or experience illusions and hallucinations.[44] Some cancer patients die suddenly, after, for example, an internal bleed. Most people decline rapidly over several days or weeks.[7]

Over this time, some people make their death a time for celebrating their life.[40] Your palliative care team, vicar, priest, pastor, rabbi, elder or other spiritual guide and counsellors can all help make death a time of 'coming together' and celebration of your life. Courage, dignity, grace and, if it's natural to you, humour can all leave a legacy that helps and inspires the next generation or two as they come to terms with the inevitable.

Putting your affairs in order

Putting your affairs in order can put your and your family's mind at rest, simplify your everyday life, help your family or friends avoid painful decisions and financial difficulties, and help you focus on your plans and goals. So, it's worth thinking about at any time in your cancer journey, even if you're in remission. You could begin by listing things you need to sort out, such as:

- making or updating your will – ideally take advice from a solicitor;
- appointing guardians for children under 18 years of age;
- listing people and organizations who should be told when you die, such as executors of your will, your employers, solicitors, financial institutions and tax authorities;
- make a list of important numbers, such as tax, pension and National Insurance;
- considering granting Power of Attorney to a family member or someone else you trust – this allows them to make decisions about your financial, legal or health affairs if you are unable to do so;
- ensuring the beneficiaries of life insurance and pension are up to date;
- listing details of all bank or building society accounts, ISAs, insurance policies, loans and credit cards, and pensions;
- creating a folder or file with important documents, such as deeds,

rent book and tenancy agreements, birth, marriage, divorce and citizenship certificates;

- listing contacts and instructions for everyday tasks that your partner may not know such as car servicing, how to use the central heating and washing machine; and so on.

Death and the carer

The death of a family member or partner from cancer can prove difficult, to say the least. You might lament the end of a close relationship. You may grieve for the relationship that you wanted and, now, can never have. Many bereaved people feel guilty that they didn't tell the person how much they loved them, how grateful they were or that they didn't apologize for something they feel guilty about.[40] Don't feel embarrassed about letting the person know how much you care.

Don't be embarrassed to grieve. Some people feel tempted to resort to drugs – legal, illegal and prescription – to blunt grief's edge. But drugs can make matters worse. Even taking anti-depressants to alleviate grief could be counterproductive. For example, almost half of people who responded to anti-depressants would not take them again because of psychological side effects including narrowing of their emotional range, not feeling themselves and an inability to cry.[126] Counselling, psychological interventions, such as guided mourning, and practical support can help. Cruse, Child Bereavement UK and your church or spiritual adviser can offer advice and support.

Complicated grief

A low mood, not feeling yourself and crying are part of normal grieving. According to one estimate, 'resolving' the loss of a loved pet means crying for at least 20 hours. 'Resolving' (you may never overcome) the loss of a spouse, parent, child or close friend requires 200–300 hours of crying.[127] Even extreme reactions are normal: about half of widows and widowers interviewed in mid-Wales reported hallucinations or illusions of their spouse.[128]

Most people begin to recover a few weeks or months after bereavement, although life will never be the same again. However, bereavement is severely stressful and triggers major depression in about one in ten people.[129, 130] Others develop debilitating 'complicated grief'. So, how can you tell the difference?

Typically, grief comes in waves and you maintain self-esteem.[75] In contrast, depression is persistent and undermines self-esteem.[131] Bereaved people are less likely to think about suicide than those with depression and are also less likely to show slowed thinking and movements, or worry excessively about past actions.[75] Nevertheless, regrets are common.

People with complicated grief, in contrast, typically endure prolonged, intense sorrow. They yearn for the deceased. They may report frequent, intrusive thoughts and memories of the deceased.[130] People with complicated grief may exhibit inappropriate behaviours and emotions. They can have difficulty comprehending the reality of the person's death or imagining a future with 'purpose and meaning'.[130]

Speak to your GP, counsellor or religious or spiritual adviser if several weeks after the death you:

• feel you have depression, PTSD (page 85) or complicated grief;
• start abusing drugs or alcohol;
• feel 'dead' or 'unreal';
• find you cannot work or take part in your normal activities.

A last word

I will leave the last word to William Osler – one of the greatest doctors in the eighteenth and early nineteenth centuries. Osler reported the case of a patient bedridden with metastatic breast cancer. The malignancy had spread to her spine, other breast and right eye. Two years later, Osler reported, 'She drove a mile and a half to the station to meet me and drove me to the station on my return.' Osler said her case – and others like it – 'are among the most remarkable' in medicine – they illustrate that 'no condition', not even cancer, 'however desperate, is quite hopeless'.[82] I wish you well.

Useful addresses

There are numerous self-help groups for specific cancers. Your cancer team or one of the charities such as Cancer Research UK or Macmillan Cancer Support should be able to put you in touch.

Action Cancer (Northern Ireland)
Action Cancer House
1 Marlborough Park
Belfast
Co. Antrim BT9 6XS
Tel.: 028 9080 3344
Website: www.actioncancer.org

Action on Smoking and Health (ASH)
Sixth Floor, Suites 59–63
New House, 67–68 Hatton Garden
London EC1N 8JY
Tel.: 020 7404 0242
Website: www.ash.org.uk

Alcohol Concern
25 Corsham Street
London N1 6DR
Tel.: 020 7566 9800
Website: www.alcoholconcern.org.uk

Alcoholics Anonymous
PO Box 1
10 Toft Green
York YO1 7NJ
Freephone Helpline: 0800 9177 650
Website: www.alcoholics-anonymous.org.uk

Ayurvedic Practitioners Association
23 Green Ridge
Brighton BN1 5LT
Tel.: 01273 470 336
Website: http://apa.uk.com

Breast Cancer Care
5–13 Great Suffolk Street
London SE1 0NS
Tel. (for advice): 0808 800 6000
(9 a.m. to 5 p.m., Monday to Friday; 5 p.m. to 7 p.m., Monday and Wednesday; 9 a.m. to 1 p.m., Saturday)
Website: www.breastcancercare.org.uk

Breast Cancer UK
BM Box 7767
London WC1N 3XX
Tel.: 0845 680 1322
Website: www.breastcanceruk.org.uk

British Association for Behavioural and Cognitive Psychotherapies
Imperial House
Hornby Street
Bury
Lancashire BL9 5BN
Tel.: 0161 705 4304
Website: www.babcp.com

British Association for Counselling and Psychotherapy
BACP House
15 St John's Business Park
Lutterworth LE17 4HB
Tel.: 01455 883300
Website: www.bacp.co.uk

British Association for Music Therapy
Second Floor, Claremont Building
24–27 White Lion Street
London N1 9PD
Tel.: 020 7837 6100
Website: www.bamt.org

British Association of Accredited
Ayurvedic Practitioners
5 Blenheim Road
North Harrow
Middlesex HA2 7AQ
Tel.: 07405 023 651
Website: www.britayurpractitioners.
com

British Association of Art
Therapists
24–27 White Lion Street
London N1 9PD
Tel.: 020 7686 4216
Website: www.baat.org

British Association of Medical
Hypnosis
45 Hyde Park Square
London W2 2JT
Website: www.bamh.org.uk

British Dietetic Association
Fifth Floor, Charles House
148/9 Great Charles Street
Queensway
Birmingham B3 3HT
Tel.: 0121 200 8080
Website: www.bda.uk.com

British Liver Trust
6 Dean Park Crescent
Bournemouth BH1 1HL
Tel.: 01425 481320
Website: www.britishlivertrust.org.uk

British Wheel of Yoga
25 Jermyn Street
Sleaford
Lincolnshire NG34 7RU
Tel.: 01529 306851
Website: www.bwy.org.uk

Cancer Research UK
Angel Building
407 St John Street
London EC1V 4AD
Tel.: 0300 123 1022
Helpline (nurses): 0808 800 4040 (9
a.m. to 5 p.m., Monday to Friday)
Website: www.cancerresearchuk.org

Child Bereavement UK
Clare Charity Centre
Wycombe Road
Saunderton
Buckinghamshire HP14 4BF
Tel.: 0800 02 888 40
Website: www.childbereavementuk.
org

Complementary and Natural
Healthcare Council
46–48 East Smithfield
London E1W 1AW
Tel.: 020 3668 0406
Website: www.cnhc.org.uk

Cruse Bereavement Care
PO Box 800
Richmond
Surrey TW9 1RG
Helpline: 0844 477 9400
Website: www.cruse.org.uk

Federation of Holistic Therapists
18 Shakespeare Business Centre
Hathaway Close
Eastleigh SO50 4SR
Tel.: 023 8062 4350
Website: www.fht.org.uk

General Regulatory Council for
Complementary Therapies
Box 437, Office 6
Slington House
Rankine Road
Basingstoke RG24 8PH
Tel.: 0870 314 4031
Website: www.grcct.org

Health and Care Professionals
Council
Park House
184 Kennington Park Road
London SE11 4BU
Tel.: 0300 500 6184
Website: www.hcpc-uk.co.uk

Institute for Complementary and
Natural Medicine (and British
Register of Complementary
Practitioners)
Can Mezzanine
32–36 Loman Street
London SE1 0EH
Tel.: 020 7922 7980
Website: http://icnm.org.uk

Leukaemia Care
One Birch Court
Blackpole East
Worcester WR3 8SG
24-hour Freephone Careline: 08088
010 444
Website: www.leukaemiacare.org.uk

Lymphoma Association
3 Cromwell Court
New Street
Aylesbury HP20 2PB
Freephone helpline: 0808 808
5555 (9 a.m. to 5 p.m., Monday to
Friday)
Website: www.lymphomas.org.uk

Macmillan Cancer Support
89 Albert Embankment
London SE1 7UQ
Helpline: 0808 808 00 00 (9 a.m. to
8 p.m., Monday to Friday)
Website: www.macmillan.org.uk

Marie Curie
89 Albert Embankment
London SE1 7TP
Support line: 0800 090 2309
Website: www.mariecurie.org.uk

National Institute of Medical
Herbalists
Clover House
James Court
South Street
Exeter EX1 1EE
Tel.: 01392 426022
Website: www.nimh.org.uk

ORCHID (male cancers)
231–233 North Gower Street
London NW1 2NR
National male cancer helpline:
0808 802 0010
Website: www.orchid-cancer.org.uk

Prostate Cancer UK
Fourth Floor, The Counting House
53 Tooley Street
London SE1 2QN
Tel.: 020 3310 7000
Website: http://prostatecanceruk.
org

Rarer Cancers Foundation
Unit 7B, Evelyn Court,
Grinstead Road,
London SE8 5AD
Helpline: 0800 334 5551 (9.30 a.m.
to 5.30 p.m., Monday to Friday)
Website: http://rarercancers.org.uk

Roy Castle Lung Cancer
Foundation
The Roy Castle Centre
4–6 Enterprise Way
Wavertree Technology Park
Liverpool L13 1FB
Tel.: 0333 323 7200
Website: www.roycastle.org

Tai Chi Union for Great Britain
Secretary
Peter Ballam
5 Corunna Drive
Horsham
West Sussex RH13 5HG
Website: www.taichiunion.com

Teenage Cancer Trust
Third Floor
93 Newman Street
London W1T 3EZ
Tel.: 020 7612 0370
Website: www.teenagecancertrust.
org

Tenovus Cancer Care
Gleider House
Ty Glas Road
Cardiff CF14 5BD
Freephone helpline: 0808 808 1010
(8 a.m. to 8 p.m., 365 days a year)
Website: www.tenovuscancercare.
org.uk

References

1   Rubin G, Berendsen A, Crawford SM, et al. The expanding role of primary care in cancer control. *The Lancet Oncology*. 2015;16:1231–72.

2   Saunders C, Jassal S. *Breast Cancer: The Facts*. Oxford University Press, 2009.

3   Brown J, Byers T, Thompson K, et al. Nutrition during and after cancer treatment: a guide for informed choices by cancer survivors. *CA: A Cancer Journal for Clinicians*. 2001;51:153–81.

4   James N. *Cancer: A Very Short Introduction*. Oxford University Press, 2011.

5   Hammer MJ, Ercolano EA, Wright F, et al. Self-management for adult patients with cancer: an integrative review. *Cancer Nursing*. 2015;38:E10–E26.

6   Priestman T. *Coping with Radiotherapy*. Sheldon Press, 2007.

7   Russell A. *The Social Basis of Medicine*. Wiley-Blackwell, 2009.

8   Schrijver K and Schrijver I. *Living with the Stars*. Oxford University Press, 2015.

9   Cancer Genome Atlas Network. Comprehensive molecular portraits of human breast tumours. *Nature*. 2012;490:61–70.

10   Cybulski C, Nazarali S, Narod SA. Multiple primary cancers as a guide to heritability. *International Journal of Cancer*. 2014;135:1756–63.

11   Madhu YC, Harish K, Gotam P. Complete resection of a giant ovarian tumour. *Gynecologic Oncology Case Reports*. 2013;6:4–6.

12   Mukherjee M. *The Emperor of All Maladies: A Biography of Cancer*. Fourth Estate, 2011.

13   Kuru B, Camlibel M, Dinc S, et al. Prognostic factors for survival in breast cancer patients who developed distant metastasis subsequent to definitive surgery. *Singapore Medical Journal*. 2008;49:904–11.

14   Matsumoto K, Oki A, Furuta R, et al. Predicting the progression of cervical precursor lesions by human papillomavirus genotyping: A prospective cohort study. *International Journal of Cancer*. 2011;128:2898–910.

15   Parkin DM, Boyd L, Walker LC. The fraction of cancer attributable to lifestyle and environmental factors in the UK in 2010. *British Journal of Cancer*. 2011;105:S77–S81.

16   Anderson TA, Schick V, Herbenick D, et al. A study of human papillomavirus on vaginally inserted sex toys, before and after cleaning, among women who have sex with women and men. *Sexually Transmitted Infections*. 2014;90:529–31.

17   King EM, Gilson R, Beddows S, et al. Oral human papillomavirus (HPV) infection in men who have sex with men: Prevalence

and lack of anogenital concordance. *Sexually Transmitted Infections.* 2015;91:284–6.

18 Hajdu SI. A note from history: Landmarks in history of cancer, part 4. *Cancer.* 2012;118:4914–28.

19 Parkin DM, Darby SC. Cancers in 2010 attributable to ionising radiation exposure in the UK. *British Journal of Cancer.* 2011;105:S57–S65.

20 Annunziato A. DNA packaging: Nucleosomes and chromatin. *Nature Education.* 2008;1:26. Available at: <www.nature.com./scitable/topicpage/dna-packaging-nucleosomes-and-chromatin-310> [accessed April 2016].

21 Friedenson B. BRCA1 and BRCA2 pathways and the risk of cancers other than breast or ovarian. *MedGenMed.* 2005;7:60.

22 Baker SG. A cancer theory kerfuffle can lead to new lines of research. *Journal of the National Cancer Institute.* 2014;107:dju405.

23 Helander HF, Fändriks L. Surface area of the digestive tract – revisited. *Scandinavian Journal of Gastroenterology.* 2014;49:681–9.

24 Badenhorst J, Husband A, Ling J, et al. Do patients with cancer alarm symptoms present at the community pharmacy? *International Journal of Pharmacy Practice.* 2014;22 (suppl 2):32.

25 Tannock IF, de Wit R, Berry WR, et al. Docetaxel plus prednisone or mitoxantrone plus prednisone for advanced prostate cancer. *New England Journal of Medicine.* 2004;351:1502–12.

26 Hirsch J. An anniversary for cancer chemotherapy. *Journal of the American Medical Association.* 2006;296:1518–20.

27 Travis LB. The epidemiology of second primary cancers. *Cancer Epidemiology Biomarkers & Prevention.* 2006;15:2020–6.

28 Anonymous. Chapter 2: The development of radiotherapy: physics, technology, methods. *Acta Oncologica.* 1996;35:24–30.

29 Anonymous. Obituary: E. H. Grubbe, MD, FACP. *British Medical Journal.* 1960;2:609.

30 Ellinger S. Micronutrients, arginine, and glutamine: Does supplementation provide an efficient tool for prevention and treatment of different kinds of wounds? *Advances in Wound Care.* 2013;3:691–707.

31 Scott A. Non-sting barrier cream in radiotherapy-induced skin reactions. *British Journal of Nursing.* 2015;24:S32, S4–7.

32 Karagöz ÖDS, Ozturk MA, Aydin Ö, et al. Receptor expression discrepancy between primary and metastatic breast cancer lesions. *Oncology Research and Treatment.* 2014;37:622–6.

33 Javier RT, Butel JS. The history of tumor virology. *Cancer Research.* 2008;68:7693–706.

34 Wu H-S, Harden JK. Symptom burden and quality of life in survivorship: A review of the literature. *Cancer Nursing.* 2015;38:E29-E54.

35 Periyakoil VS, Neri E, Kraemer H. Patient-reported barriers to high-quality, end-of-life care: A multiethnic, multilingual, mixed-methods study. *Journal of Palliative Medicine.* 2016;19(4):373–9.

36 Komatsu H, Yagasaki K, Yamauchi H, et al. A self-directed home

yoga programme for women with breast cancer during chemotherapy: A feasibility study. *International Journal of Nursing Practice*. 2015:DOI:10.1111/ijn.12419.

37 Atkins L, Fallowfield L. Intentional and non-intentional non-adherence to medication amongst breast cancer patients. *European Journal of Cancer*. 2006;42:2271–6.

38 Brown J, Byers T, Thompson K, et al. Nutrition during and after cancer treatment: A guide for informed choices by cancer survivors. *CA: A Cancer Journal for Clinicians*. 2001;51:153–81.

39 Durdu Keskin O, Kertmen N, Karakas Y, et al. A systemic late recurrence after the first operation in a patient diagnosed with early-stage breast cancer: The latest recurrence in the literature. *Journal of Balkan Union of Oncology*. 2015;20:348.

40 Chochinov H, Breitbart W (eds). *Handbook of Psychiatry in Palliative Medicine*, second edition. Oxford University Press, 2009.

41 Watson M, Haviland JS, Greer S, et al. Influence of psychological response on survival in breast cancer: A population-based cohort study. *The Lancet*. 1999;354:1331–6.

42 Watson M, Homewood J, Haviland J, et al. Influence of psychological response on breast cancer survival: 10-year follow-up of a population-based cohort. *European Journal of Cancer*. 2005;41:1710–4.

43 Parkin DM, Boyd L. Cancers attributable to overweight and obesity in the UK in 2010. *British Journal of Cancer*. 2011;105:S34–S37.

44 Newton S, Hickey M, Marrs J. *Mosby's Oncology Nursing Advisor: A Comprehensive Guide to Clinical Practice*. Mosby, 2009.

45 Hofbauer K, Anker S, Inui A, et al. *Pharmacotherapy of Cachexia*. CRC Press, 2005.

46 Yang M, Kenfield SA, Van Blarigan EL, et al. Dietary patterns after prostate cancer diagnosis in relation to disease-specific and total mortality. *Cancer Prevention Research*. 2015;8:545–51.

47 Kenfield SA, Batista JL, Jahn JL, et al. Development and application of a lifestyle score for prevention of lethal prostate cancer. *Journal of the National Cancer Institute*. 2016;108 (3): djv329.

48 Norat T, Aune D, Chan D, et al. Fruits and vegetables: Updating the epidemiologic evidence for the WCRF/AICR lifestyle recommendations for cancer prevention. In: Zappia V, Panico S, Russo LG, Budillon A, Della Ragione F (eds). *Advances in Nutrition and Cancer*. Springer Berlin Heidelberg, 2014. p.35–50.

49 Oyebode O, Gordon-Dseagu V, Walker A, et al. Fruit and vegetable consumption and all-cause, cancer and CVD mortality: Analysis of Health Survey for England data. *Journal of Epidemiology and Community Health*. 2014;68:856–62.

50 Aune D, Chan DSM, Lau R, et al. Dietary fibre, whole grains, and risk of colorectal cancer: Systematic review and dose-response meta-analysis of prospective studies. *British Medical Journal*. 2011;343:d6617.

51 Tektonidis TG, Akesson A, Gigante B, et al. A Mediterranean diet and

risk of myocardial infarction, heart failure and stroke: A population-based cohort study. *Atherosclerosis*. 2015;243:93–8.

52   Challier B, Perarnau JM, Viel JF. Garlic, onion and cereal fibre as protective factors for breast cancer: A French case-control study. *European Journal of Epidemiology*. 1998;14:737–47.

53   Cade JE, Burley VJ, Greenwood DC. Dietary fibre and risk of breast cancer in the UK Women's Cohort Study. *International Journal of Epidemiology*. 2007;36:431–8.

54   Armstrong LE, Ganio MS, Casa DJ, et al. Mild dehydration affects mood in healthy young women. *The Journal of Nutrition*. 2012;142:382–8.

55   Ganio MS, Armstrong LE, Casa DJ, et al. Mild dehydration impairs cognitive performance and mood of men. *British Journal of Nutrition*. 2011;106:1535–43.

56   Nestle M. Mediterranean diets: Historical and research overview. *The American Journal of Clinical Nutrition*. 1995;61:1313S–20S.

57   Toledo E, Salas-Salvadó J, Donat-Vargas C, et al. Mediterranean diet and invasive breast cancer risk among women at high cardiovascular risk in the predimed trial: A randomized clinical trial. *JAMA Internal Medicine*. 2015:1–9.

58   Zhang M, Huang J, Xie X, et al. Dietary intakes of mushrooms and green tea combine to reduce the risk of breast cancer in Chinese women. *International Journal of Cancer*. 2009;124:1404–8.

59   Han C-K, Chiang H-C, Lin C-Y, et al. Comparison of immunomodulatory and anticancer activities in different strains of *Tremella fuciformis* berk. *The American Journal of Chinese Medicine*. 2015;43:1637–55.

60   Paterson RR, Lima N. Biomedical effects of mushrooms with emphasis on pure compounds. *Biomedical Journal*. 2014;37:357–68.

61   Fritz H, Kennedy DA, Ishii M, et al. Polysaccharide K and *Coriolus versicolor* extracts for lung cancer: A systematic review. *Integrative Cancer Therapies*. 2015;14:201–11.

62   Bettuzzi S, Brausi M, Rizzi F, et al. Chemoprevention of human prostate cancer by oral administration of green tea catechins in volunteers with high-grade prostate intraepithelial neoplasia: A preliminary report from a one-year proof-of-principle study. *Cancer Research*. 2006;66:1234–40.

63   Simopoulos AP. The traditional diet of Greece and cancer. *European Journal of Cancer Prevention*. 2004;13:219–30.

64   Murphy RA, Mourtzakis M, Chu QSC, et al. Supplementation with fish oil increases first-line chemotherapy efficacy in patients with advanced nonsmall cell lung cancer. *Cancer*. 2011;117:3774–80.

65   Murphy RA, Mourtzakis M, Chu QSC, et al. Nutritional intervention with fish oil provides a benefit over standard of care for weight and skeletal muscle mass in patients with nonsmall cell lung cancer receiving chemotherapy. *Cancer*. 2011;117:1775–82.

66   Ben-Arye E, Polliack A, Schiff E, et al. Advising patients on the use of non-herbal nutritional supplements during cancer therapy: A

need for doctor-patient communication. *Journal of Pain and Symptom Management*. 2013;46:887–96.

67 NICE. *Vitamin D: Increasing supplement use among at-risk groups*. Available at: <www.nice.org.uk/guidance/ph56> [accessed April 2016].

68 Holick MF. Vitamin D deficiency. *New England Journal of Medicine*. 2007;357:266–81.

69 NIH (National Institutes of Health). *Office of Dietary Supplements – Vitamin D*. 2016. Available at: <https://ods.od.nih.gov/factsheets/VitaminD-HealthProfessional/> [accessed April 2016].

70 Kravits KG. Hypnosis for the management of anticipatory nausea and vomiting. *Journal of the Advanced Practitioner in Oncology*. 2015;6:225–9.

71 Malton S. Managing chemo side-effects. *Pharmacy Magazine*. 2015;June:16.

72 Sutton A, Crew A, Wysong A. Redefinition of skin cancer as a chronic disease. *JAMA Dermatology*. 2016;152(3):255.

73 Dautricourt S, Marzloff V, Dollfus S. Meningiomatosis revealed by a major depressive syndrome. *BMJ Case Reports*. 2015;DOI:10.1136/bcr-2015-211909.

74 Tylee A, Gandhi P. The importance of somatic symptoms in depression in primary care. *The Primary Care Companion for CNS Disorders*. 2005;7:167–76.

75 Edwards V. *Depression: What you really need to know*. Robinson, 2003.

76 Russell A. *The Social Basis of Medicine*, first edition. Wiley Blackwell, 2009.

77 Hoge EA, Ivkovic A, Fricchione GL. Generalized anxiety disorder: Diagnosis and treatment. *British Medical Journal*. 2012;345:e7500

78 Wachen JS, Patidar SM, Mulligan EA, et al. Cancer-related PTSD symptoms in a veteran sample: Association with age, combat PTSD, and quality of life. *Psycho-Oncology*. 2014;23:921–7.

79 Liao Y-H, Lin C-C, Lai H-C, et al. Adjunctive traditional Chinese medicine therapy improves survival of liver cancer patients. *Liver International*. 2015;135:2595–602)

80 Lee Y-W, Chen T-L, Shih Y-RV, et al. Adjunctive traditional Chinese medicine therapy improves survival in patients with advanced breast cancer: A population-based study. *Cancer*. 2014;120:1338–44.

81 Wall P. Pain and the placebo response. *Ciba Foundation Symposium*. 1993;174:187–211; discussion 212–6.

82 Papac R. Spontaneous regression of cancer. *Cancer Treatment Reviews*. 1996;22:395–423.

83 Ventegodt S, Jacobsen S, Merrick J. Clinical holistic medicine: A case of induced spontaneous remission in a patient with non-Hodgkin b-lymphoma. *Journal of Alternative Medcine Research*. 2009;1:101–10.

84 Vickers AJ, Cronin AM, Maschino AC, et al. Acupuncture for chronic pain: Individual patient data meta-analysis. *Archives of Internal Medicine*. 2012;172:1444–53.

85   Pachman DR, Price KA, Carey EC. Nonpharmacologic approach to fatigue in patients with cancer. *The Cancer Journal*. 2014;20:313–8.

86   Lehrner J, Eckersberger C, Walla P, et al. Ambient odor of orange in a dental office reduces anxiety and improves mood in female patients. *Physiology & Behavior*. 2000;71:83–6.

87   Kirsch I. *The Emperor's New Drugs: Exploding the antidepressant myth*. Bodley Head, 2009.

88   Bivins R. *Alternative Medicine? A history*. Oxford University Press, 2007.

89   Montgomery GH, Schnur JB, Kravits K. Hypnosis for cancer care: Over 200 years young. *CA: A Cancer Journal for Clinicians*. 2013; 63:31–44.

90   Chen Y-W, Hunt MA, Campbell KL, et al. The effect of Tai Chi on four chronic conditions – cancer, osteoarthritis, heart failure and chronic obstructive pulmonary disease: A systematic review and meta-analyses. *British Journal of Sports Medicine*. 2015;50(7):397–407.

91   Renneberg R. Biotech history: Yew trees, paclitaxel synthesis and fungi. *Biotechnology Journal*. 2007;2:1207–9.

92   Newman DJ, Cragg GM. Natural products as sources of new drugs over the 30 years from 1981 to 2010. *Journal of Natural Products*. 2012;75:311–35.

93   Marvibaigi M, Supriyanto E, Amini N, et al. Preclinical and clinical effects of mistletoe against breast cancer. *BioMed Research International*. 2014;2014:15.

94   Abenavoli L, Capasso R, Milic N, et al. Milk thistle in liver diseases: Past, present, future. *Phytotherapy Research*. 2010;24:1423–32.

95   Chang S-M, Chen C-H. Effects of an intervention with drinking chamomile tea on sleep quality and depression in sleep disturbed postnatal women: A randomized controlled trial. *Journal of Advanced Nursing*. 2016;72:306–15.

96   Xu Y, Chen Y, Li P, et al. *Ren Shen Yangrong Tang* for fatigue in cancer survivors: a phase I/II open-label study. *The Journal of Alternative and Complementary Medicine*. 2015;21:281–7.

97   Lin H-C, Lin C-L, Huang W-Y, et al. The use of adjunctive traditional Chinese medicine therapy and survival outcome in patients with head and neck cancer: A nationwide population-based cohort study. *QJM*. 2015; 108 (12):959–65.

98   Cassileth BR, Vickers AJ. Massage therapy for symptom control: Outcome study at a major cancer center. *Journal of Pain and Symptom Management*. 2004;28:244–9.

99   Taylor AG, Snyder AE, Anderson JG, et al. Gentle massage improves disease- and treatment-related symptoms in patients with acute myelogenous leukemia. *Journal of Clinical Trials*. 2014. DOI:10.4172/2167-0870.1000161.

100   Johns S, Von Ah D, Brown L, et al. Randomized controlled pilot trial of mindfulness-based stress reduction for breast and colorectal cancer survivors: Effects on cancer-related cognitive impairment. *Journal of Cancer Survivorship*. 2016; 10:437–48.

101   Gould J. Mental health: Stressed students reach out for help. *Nature*. 2014;512:223–4.

102   Streeter CC, Whitfield TH, Owen L, et al. Effects of yoga versus walking on mood, anxiety, and brain GABA levels: A randomized controlled MRS study. *The Journal of Alternative and Complementary Medicine*. 2010;16:1145–52.

103   DeBoer LB, Powers MB, Utschig AC, et al. Exploring exercise as an avenue for the treatment of anxiety disorders. *Expert Review of Neurotherapeutics*. 2012;12:1011–22.

104   Pan Y, Yang K, Wang Y, et al. Could yoga practice improve treatment-related side effects and quality of life for women with breast cancer? A systematic review and meta-analysis. *Asia-Pacific Journal of Clinical Oncology*. 2015; DOI:10.1111/ajco.12329.

105   Parkin DM. Tobacco-attributable cancer burden in the UK in 2010. *British Journal of Cancer*. 2011;105:S6–S13.

106   Danson S, Rowland C, Rowe R, et al. The relationship between smoking and quality of life in advanced lung cancer patients: A prospective longitudinal study. *Supportive Care in Cancer*. 2015:1–10.

107   Baser S, Shannon VR, Eapen GA, et al. Smoking cessation after diagnosis of lung cancer is associated with a beneficial effect on performance status. *Chest*. 2006;130:1784–90.

108   Semple S, Apsley A, Azmina Ibrahim T, et al. Fine particulate matter concentrations in smoking households: Just how much secondhand smoke do you breathe in if you live with a smoker who smokes indoors? *Tobacco Control*. 2014;24(e3):e205-e211.

109   Clancy N, Zwar N, Richmond R. Depression, smoking and smoking cessation: A qualitative study. *Family Practice*. 2013;30:587–92.

110   Miller PM, Day TA, Ravenel MC. Clinical implications of continued alcohol consumption after diagnosis of upper aerodigestive tract cancer. *Alcohol and Alcoholism*. 2006;41:140–2.

111   Nelson DE, Jarman DW, Rehm J, et al. Alcohol-attributable cancer deaths and years of potential life lost in the United States. *American Journal of Public Health*. 2013;103:641–8.

112   Battaglini CL, Mills RC, Phillips BL, et al. Twenty-five years of research on the effects of exercise training in breast cancer survivors: A systematic review of the literature. *World Journal of Clinical Oncology*. 2014;5:177–90.

113   Borch KB, Braaten T, Lund E, et al. Physical activity before and after breast cancer diagnosis and survival – the Norwegian women and cancer cohort study. *BMC Cancer*. 2015;15:1–10.

114   Otto M, Smits J. *Exercise for Mood and Anxiety: Proven strategies for overcoming depression and enhancing well-being*. Oxford University Press, 2011.

115   Ulrich R. View through a window may influence recovery from surgery. *Science*. 1984;224:420–1.

116   Park B, Tsunetsugu Y, Kasetani T, et al. The physiological effects of *Shinrin-yoku* (taking in the forest atmosphere or forest bathing):

Evidence from field experiments in 24 forests across Japan. *Environmental Health and Preventative Medicine.* 2010;15:18–26.

117 Takayama N, Korpela K, Lee J, et al. Emotional, restorative and vitalizing effects of forest and urban environments at four sites in Japan. *International Journal of Environmental Research and Public Health.* 2014;11:7207–30.

118 Phelps C, Butler C, Cousins A, et al. Sowing the seeds or failing to blossom? A feasibility study of a simple ecotherapy-based intervention in women affected by breast cancer. *ecancer.* 2015;6:602.

119 Fingelkurts AA. Is our brain hardwired to produce God, or is our brain hardwired to perceive God? A systematic review on the role of the brain in mediating religious experience. *Cognitive Processing.* 2009;10:293–326.

120 Polkinghorne J. *Exploring Reality.* SPCK, 2005.

121 Jim HSL, Pustejovsky JE, Park CL, et al. Religion, spirituality, and physical health in cancer patients: A meta-analysis. *Cancer.* 2015;121:3760–8.

122 Burkhart L, Schmidt L, Hogan N. Development and psychometric testing of the Spiritual Care Inventory instrument. *Journal of Advanced Nursing.* 2011;67:2463–72.

123 Park C, Dornelas E. Is religious coping related to better quality of life following acute myocardial infarction? *Journal of Religion and Health.* 2012;51:1337–46.

124 Ong AD, Bergeman CS, Boker SM. Resilience comes of age: Defining features in later adulthood. *Journal of Personality.* 2009;77:1777–804.

125 Matuszek S. Animal-facilitated therapy in various patient populations: Systematic literature review. *Holistic Nursing Practice.* 2010;24:187–203.

126 Antonuccio D, Healy D. Relabeling the medications we call antidepressants. *Scientifica.* 2012;2012:965908.

127 Dugan DO. Laughter and tears: Best medicine for stress. *Nursing Forum.* 1989;24:18–26.

128 Dewi Rees W. The hallucinations of widowhood. *British Medical Journal.* 1971;4:37–41.

129 American Psychiatric Association *Diagnostic and Statistical Manual of Mental Disorders,* fifth edition. Washington, DC, 2013.

130 Shear M, Wang Y, Skritskaya N, et al. Treatment of complicated grief in elderly persons: A randomized clinical trial. *JAMA Psychiatry.* 2014;71:1287–95.

131 Bower B. DSM-5 enters the diagnostic fray: Fifth edition of the widely used psychiatric manual focuses attention on how mental disorders should be defined. *Science News.* 2013;183:5–6.

132 McDonnell SL, Baggerly C, French CB, Baggerly LL, Garland CF, et al. Serum 25-Hydroxyvitamin D concentrations ≥40 ng/ml are associated with >65% lower cancer risk: Pooled analysis of randomized trial and prospective cohort study. *PLoS ONE.* 2016; 11(4): e0152441.

Further reading

Ausubel, Kenny. *When Healing Becomes a Crime: The amazing story of the Hoxsey Cancer Clinics and the return of alternative therapies*. Healing Arts Press, 2000.

Blythe, Ronald. *From the Headlands*. Chatto & Windus, 1982.

Freeman, Jane. *How to Eat Well When You Have Cancer*. Sheldon Press, 2012.

Geiger, Chris. *The Cancer Survivors Club: A collection of inspirational and uplifting stories*. Oneworld Publications, 2015.

Greener, Mark. *Coping with Liver Disease*. Sheldon Press, 2013.

Greener, Mark. *Coping with Thyroid Disease*. Sheldon Press, 2014.

Greener, Mark. *Depression and Anxiety the Drug-Free Way*. Sheldon Press, 2015.

Greener, Mark. *The Holistic Health Handbook*. Sheldon Press, 2013.

James, Nicholas. *Cancer: A very short introduction*. Oxford University Press, 2011.

Krementsov, Nikolai. *The Cure: A story of cancer and politics from the annals of the Cold War*. University of Chicago Press, 2004.

Mukherjee, Siddhartha. *The Emperor of All Maladies: A biography of cancer*. Fourth Estate, 2011.

Shaw, Clare. *The Royal Marsden Cancer Cookbook*. Kyle Books, 2015.

Solzhenitsyn, Alexander. *Cancer Ward*. Vintage Classics, 2003.

Sontag, Susan. *Illness as Metaphor and AIDS and Its Metaphors*. Penguin Modern Classics, 2009.

Styron, William. *Darkness Visible: A memoir of madness*. Jonathan Cape, 1991.

Tugendhat, Julia. *How to Approach Death*. Sheldon Press, 2007.

Index

143